Penguin Books
Meditation for Everybody

Louis Proto is the author of *The Feeling Good Book* (1983),
Coming Alive (1987), *Take Charge of Your Life* (1988), *Who's
Pulling Your Strings?* (1989), *Total Relaxation in Five Steps:
The Alpha Plan* (Penguin 1989) *Self-Healing* (1990) and
Increase Your Energy (1991). A graduate of London
University and a Westminster Pastoral Foundation-trained
psychotherapist, he brings to his work with individuals and
groups his experience over the last twenty years of both
Eastern and Western methods of facilitating awareness,
personal growth and relaxation. Eclectic in approach, he
draws on a variety of sources such as holistic therapies, zen,
yoga and meditation (which he practised for three years in
India) and in his books has made these techniques for well-
being and relaxation available to a much wider public. His
unique approach has attracted the interest of the national
press, and he has regularly been interviewed on radio and
answered listeners' questions.

LOUIS PROTO

MEDITATION
FOR
EVERYBODY

PENGUIN BOOKS

PENGUIN BOOKS

Published by the Penguin Group
Penguin Books Ltd, 27 Wrights Lane, London W8 5TZ, England
Penguin Books USA Inc., 375 Hudson Street, New York, New York 10014, USA
Penguin Books Australia Ltd, Ringwood, Victoria, Australia
Penguin Books Canada Ltd, 10 Alcorn Avenue, Toronto, Ontario, Canada M4V 3B2
Penguin Books (NZ) Ltd, 182–190 Wairau Road, Auckland 10, New Zealand

Penguin Books Ltd, Registered Offices: Harmondsworth, Middlesex, England

First published 1991
10 9 8 7 6 5 4 3 2

The ten woodcuts on pp. 37–8 first appeared in *Zen Flesh, Zen Bones* by Paul Reps.
copyright © The Charles E. Tuttle Co., Inc., 1957. Reprinted by permission The Charles
E. Tuttle Co., Inc.
The Chakras illustration on p. 98 represents The Body–Mirror System, copyright ©
Martin Brofman. Reproduced by permission Martin Brofman.

The moral right of the author has been asserted

Printed in England by Clays Ltd, St Ives plc
Filmset in Melior

Acknowledgements

My thanks are due to Isabel Maxwell Cade for allowing me to reproduce the diagrams of Alpha and Beta brainwaves and to Martin Brofman for the chart of the chakras. And, finally, to all the Masters, teachers of meditation, and friends who made this book possible, and to whom it is dedicated.

Contents

Meditation Techniques

Introduction:
MEDITATION FOR EVERYBODY

As the person becomes integrated so does his world.
As he feels good, so does the world look good.
Abraham Maslow

For Clint Eastwood it's 'a way of recharging my batteries'. Tina Turner insists that it was meditation that helped her build up her self-confidence again after her emotionally – and physically – bruising marriage to former partner Ike and contributed to her success in a new career as a solo performer. Burt Reynolds, somewhat mysteriously, tells us 'it saved my life'.

Shirley Ann Field began meditating five years ago.

> Within a few months the asthma I've had since I
> was a child cleared up. I found myself becoming
> calmer, more in control of situations, not so 'thrown'
> by things that came up. But the best thing has
> been that these days I don't suffer so much from
> stage fright. Ever since I started out as an actress
> in the 1950s I've been paralysed by fear before a
> performance. Sometimes I would even come out in
> a rash. Now I still of course get 'keyed up' before
> going on stage – but only normally so. Meditating
> every day has made an enormous improvement in
> the quality of my life.

Some other stars who have revealed in interviews that they are regular meditators include: Bruce Springsteen, Diana Ross, George Harrison, Larry Hagman, Stephanie Beacham,

Stevie Wonder, Richard Gere, Rupert Everett and Sandie Shaw.

A popular form of meditation among show business people would seem to be chanting. Peter Dean (who plays stallholder Pete in 'EastEnders') swears by it. A practising Buddhist, he chants both morning and evening and says that it has helped him to become 'a happier, healthier and generally nicer human being'. Boy George claims that chanting helped him unhook himself from heroin.

It is not so surprising that people in a profession whose uncertainty and pressures have resulted in so many tragic casualities in the past (one thinks of Billie Holiday, Garland, Monroe, Janis Joplin, Brian Jones, Hendrix) have turned to meditation as a way of unwinding and staying on an even keel. It's healthier than tranquillizers or alcohol – and a lot cheaper.

But the benefits of meditation go beyond merely helping us relax, keeping us in balance and more able to cope with pressures. Paradoxically, learning how to switch off our minds when we are not using them makes them more efficient when we switch them on again. Meditation makes for clarity, improved concentration and effectiveness at work. It is for this reason that the best-known form of meditation in the West (Transcendental Meditation®) has been recommended by business corporations in the USA for their executives and employees. It makes for improved efficiency and more harmonious relations within organizations.

Since the days when The Beatles played a key role in 'bringing' meditation to the West by their highly publicized connection with the Maharishi in the sixties, meditation has gradually been assimilated into our culture; in other words, it is becoming 'ordinary'. Twenty years on it has been 'lifted' from the eastern religious matrix which formed it, and rescued from exclusive association with hippies and flower children. Today you don't have to be a Buddhist or Hindu (or, indeed, 'religious' at all), a seeker after enlightenment or a 'freak' hooked on cosmic experiences, in order to meditate. You may simply be so fed up with being pushed around by your mind and being over-stressed that you are willing to explore what you can do about it, keen to learn how to unwind, switch off the outside world and its clamour and relax into yourself. For this is all meditation is – returning home after being out in the market-place, relaxing and feeling again who you are. And who you are is not your mind.

1
DON'T LET YOUR MIND DRIVE YOU CRAZY!

Walk or sit. But don't wobble.

Zen saying

ARE YOU
an obsessive worrier?
unable to switch off after you've finished work?
finding it hard to relax and enjoy yourself?
workaholic?
restless?
tense?
constantly 'on the go', finding things to do?
dissatisfied without knowing why?
easily bored when there's nothing happening?
living in the past?
living for the future?
unable to concentrate?
at the mercy of your moods?
feeling insecure?
feeling in a rut?
looking for a new direction?

OUTER STRESS – INNER STRESS
Judging by the number of books on stress and stress management, we have got the message that we should learn how to slow down and take things a lot easier if we are to stay in good health. The list of stress-related diseases lengthens as medical research explores the deleterious effects on our

bodies of daily exposure to noise, speed, pollution, and the pressures of earning a living in an expensive and competitive world. We know now all about the 'fight or flight' response to stressful situations, the damage done to our immune systems by the continual release of adrenalin and cortico-steroids in response to these situations, the higher risk of having a coronary if we are Type A (particularly competitive, workaholic, goal-orientated and time-pressured). Accordingly, many people are now incorporating into their lives activities that help to discharge the tensions of the working day (e.g. jogging), and learning techniques for relaxation (e.g. auto-genics) – and this is good.

But merely to exercise and relax the body is not enough. As Hans Selye pointed out in his trail-blazing work *The Stress of Life* thirty years ago, it is the stress that we generate *from within ourselves* that is far more dangerous than anything that can come at us from the outside. The new science of psychoimmunology is revealing just how much our bodies are affected by what goes on in our minds, for better or for worse. Unrelieved worrying, harbouring resentment, mourning loss for too long are mind patterns that have been linked with the onset of cancer in several studies. Long-standing anxiety, low self-image and a sense of insecurity – or 'victim consciousness' – is now being suspected as contributing to AIDS, the burn-out of an immune system forced to be constantly on 'red alert'.

It really is important to learn to take charge of our minds if we are to enjoy quality as well as good health in our lives. Our lives are stressful enough as it is without adding to the stress from within. Learning how to switch off the mind's activity temporarily by deeply relaxing for a period every day is one of the healthiest things we can do for ourselves, for it repairs the daily wear and tear on our nervous systems, recharges our batteries, strengthens our immune systems and is prophylactic against stress disease. Not only that, but getting some relief from the stranglehold of our minds is deeply satisfying.

Meditation is the time-honoured way of controlling the mind. And in these *angst*-ridden times there has never been such a need for it.

THE MIND MACHINE

Everybody has the same problem. It is called 'Mind'. That may surprise you. You may be proud of your mind, how you can hold your own in any argument, come up with the right answers at conferences at work, finish the *Daily Telegraph* crossword in your lunch-hour. You may have spent a lot of time and effort at school and university developing your mind's faculties of logic, analysis, memory, which now enable you to earn your living. And, since you are constantly being rewarded and achieving recognition for the cleverness of your mind, it is not surprising that you have come to be identified with it, to assume that you *are* your mind, rather than, as is the case, that it is the instrument with which you make sense of the world around you.

Mind's ability to conceptualize, to discriminate between options, to plan ahead, to verbalize and manipulate language so as to communicate the finest shades of meaning has made us the dominant species on this planet. Mind has enabled us to rule the world, and to transform it with our endless capacity for invention. The cities in which we live, our homes full of artefacts and machines that are themselves the off-spring of the minds that engineered them – all originated initially as *ideas* in the minds of city planners, government departments officials, designers, architects, and so forth. Our leisure moments are spent enjoying the mind creations of others: a novel, perhaps, the latest Spielberg or James Bond film, or just what happens to be on the television. We are sur-rounded by Mind, it is the *milieu* in which we live.

So what is the problem? The problem is that in our

eagerness to evolve our mind machines to their utmost potential we omitted to learn how to switch them off when they were not needed, rather like a blaring radio whose control knob has come off in our hands. Or like the computer in Kubrick's *2001* that has ideas above its station and ends up taking over the space craft, to general alarm and despondency; it no longer serves its masters as a source of ready information when needed nor shuts up when told to. Like Dr Frankenstein's famous creation, when our minds get out of control and 'do their own thing' they can be, at the very least, a pain in the neck, and, at worst, monsters. They can make us, at best, uncomfortable, tense, restless, unable to relax and enjoy, and, at worst, ill, criminal or insane. What, after all, is neurosis but our mind's persecution of us, and psychosis, but its running amok?

To meditate is to experience relief from the mind's constant restlessness and chatter and to feel silent and at peace within. There are many ways to achieve this, and this book suggests meditation techniques — 'ways in' to this inner peace — that you might like to experiment with to see which best suit you.

THE THINKER NOT THE THOUGHT

Really, 'mind' as an entity does not exist. If we observe, there is only a stream of consciousness, a procession of thoughts that is more or less automatic. These thoughts arise like bubbles out of nowhere. Some are agreeable to us, some disagreeable, some neutral in feeling content. Sometimes they disappear again almost immediately, sometimes they persist in remaining in our awareness, clamouring for our attention or action, haunting, if not actually persecuting us. Since feeling follows thought, they can make us feel anything from happy, satisfied or euphoric to depressed, desperate or paranoid.

These thoughts that come willy-nilly into our heads affect

our moods, and, since what we say and do usually arises from what we are feeling, they affect our actions and reactions to others as well. Our thoughts therefore manipulate us as surely as puppets on a string. When one thought takes us over, we feel sexy; another (perhaps of the tax money now due that we have already spent), we panic. Remembering old hurts, we feel the same old anger coming up, just as if it was happening all over again. In the midst of a celebration or other occasion meant to be fun we can suddenly be brought down by an *angst*-laden thought and reminded of our problems – and our joy flies out of the window. Our thoughts *drive* us: up and down we go, round and round, for all the world like mice on a treadmill.

The greatest insights of the East have been into the nature of mind – that it is at the root of all human unhappiness, simply because everything starts as a thought before being acted on and being manifested on the material plane. And the greatest contribution of the East to human happiness has been meditation – the only way to cut through the stranglehold our thought process has on our experience and way of being in the world.

The essence of 'getting off the wheel' is to break the identification of ourselves with our thoughts, to become less robot-like and driven by them. To realize (as one does with regular meditation) that one is the *thinker* of thoughts rather than the thoughts themselves, the container not the content, is tremendously liberating. One gets to realize that one does not *have* to be disturbed by whatever disaster movie is at the moment being projected onto the mind screen, by gloom-laden memories of the past or doom-laden fantasies of the future. Problems may remain, but they now become *facts* that have to be handled – and they will be handled more efficiently if they can be seen clearly rather than through the fog of feelings that usually clusters around them. Meditation allows us to see what is real more clearly, to experience it more directly, to respond to it more appropriately *as it is now*, undistracted by what our minds are telling us about what might or should happen, or what happened last time. For our minds are never in the here and now, but dwelling in the past or the future. Perhaps the greatest thing regular meditation does for us is to increase our capacity for living in the moment and therefore heightening our experience of what is happening to us. It really does help us to 'lose our minds and come to our senses' – which is another way of saying it makes us feel more alive, more truly 'here'.

WHAT REGULAR MEDITATION CAN DO FOR YOU

PHYSICAL BENEFITS:

decreases tension
clears up psychosomatic ailments caused by tension
prophylactic against stress disease
lowers blood pressure
strengthens immune system
slows down the ageing process
recharges batteries.

PSYCHOLOGICAL BENEFITS:

calms
soothes
energizes
distances from worries
integrates
brings clarity
enhances sense of self
promotes personal growth.

AT WORK:

better concentration
less capacity for being distracted

improved memory
quicker learning (e.g. languages)
staying centred under pressure
facilitates flow of creative ideas.

AT PLAY:

heightened enjoyment through the senses
present-centredness
capacity for total involvement
non-seriousness.

IN RELATING:

more self-confidence
more tolerance
more sensitivity
more authenticity.

There have been about 350 scientific studies carried out into the effects of regular meditation. The following is a short list of these effects as discovered by the Transcendental Meditation® research programme.

DEVELOPMENT OF MENTAL POTENTIAL:

optimization of brain functioning
broader comprehension and improved ability to focus
development of creativity
development of intelligence
more learning ability.

BENEFITS FOR EDUCATION:

increased academic achievement
improved academic performance in university students.

IMPROVEMENTS IN HEALTH:

more efficient physiological functioning

more effective interaction with the environment
beneficial effects on bronchial asthma
less chance of heart attacks
younger looks
improved health and longevity in the elderly
reduced need for medical care
decreased incidence of disease.

IMPROVEMENTS IN SOCIAL BEHAVIOUR:
improved self-image
development of personality
speedier recovery from stress
reduced use of caffeine, tobacco, alcohol, drugs.

BENEFITS FOR BUSINESS AND INDUSTRY:
increased productivity
improved relations at work
increased physiological relaxation and decreased stress
better health
improved job performance, job satisfaction and relationships.*

It is amazing (but true) that so many good things can happen merely by 'sitting quietly, doing nothing' (which is how meditation practice is described in zen). We have been conditioned to think that the only way we can improve our quality of life is by working harder, making more effort (remember those school reports?), by *doing* more. But meditation is a *non-doing*, and is about effortlessness. In fact you cannot *do* meditation at all: you can only *relax* into it, and allow it to happen. It is a surrendering to what 'is', rather than trying to control the way things 'should be'. It is in this surrender, this relinquishment of the compulsive urge to 'do', that meditation brings us to the deepest level of

* *Scientific Research on the Maharishi Technology of the Unified Field: The Transcendental Meditation and TM-Sidhi Program*, Maharishi International University, 1988.

psychophysical relaxation possible this side of sleep. It is the relaxation technique *par excellence*, for it is the only way to relax not only the body, but the mind. And without a relaxed mind we can never be *totally* relaxed. 'Just resting' and sometimes – for example, if we are tense through worry – even sleeping do not go deep enough.

WHAT HAPPENS WHEN WE MEDITATE?

When we meditate we let go of the 'fight or flight response' (associated with anger or anxiety) and sink into the 'relaxation response': breathing slows, heart rate and blood pressure lower, muscles relax. There is also a decrease of blood lactate and an increase in the skin's resistance to a mild electric current – significant because lactic acid concentration in the blood is associated with anxiety states. Also, when people are anxious they tend to perspire more, which decreases skin resistance to an electric current. (This can be measured by special machines, and is the principle behind the lie-detector.) In short, our tension evaporates as we slow down, unwind, 'switch off' during our meditation session.

But what, you may be asking yourself, is the difference between that and what happens when I just put my feet up and relax, or take a nap? The answer is that the decrease in metabolic rate (using up oxygen and producing carbon dioxide) happens much faster when you are meditating than when you are sleeping. During meditation the rate of decrease of oxygen consumption averages between 10 and 20 per cent and occurs within a few minutes of starting to meditate. When we are asleep, on the other hand, our consumption of oxygen decreases only slowly. After four or five hours it is still only about 8 per cent lower than when we were awake. Also, lactate concentration in the blood decreases during meditation almost four times as quickly as it does if you are just 'putting your feet up', while skin resistance has been found in some cases to increase as much as 400 per cent.

Changes happen in brainwave activity during meditation which are quite different from 'just resting' or sleep patterns. These have been measured using an electroencephalograph (usually abbreviated to EEG) or some form of biofeedback such as C. Maxwell Cade's *Mind Mirror* (see below). We spend most of our working day (and perhaps most of our waking state) functioning on the Beta wavelength. This means that the electrical activity in our brains is varying within the range of between 14 and 26 times per second (usually measured as cycles per second, indicated by the symbol Hz). If we are having a hard day at the office we will be high on the Beta scale rather than low, because the greater the effort or stress, the higher, the faster the frequency. Beta is our 'everyday mind', associated with thinking, planning, doing, concentrating, problem-solving and generally focusing upon the outside world and meeting its demands. The Beta state is not a particularly unpleasant or uncomfortable state to be in (except perhaps on a rainy Monday morning queueing to get the bus to work – and especially if you're late) providing you don't go too high in it – or stay too long in it without 'coming down' (i.e. relaxing in some way).

What happens, then, when we relax is that our brainwaves slow down to the lower frequency of 8 to 13 Hz that we call Alpha. Just as Beta waves are associated with 'being on the go', so the Alpha state is experienced as feelings of wellbeing – particularly of 'having space' i.e. not being under pressure. The more we relax, the deeper we go into the Alpha state. If we slow down even more (below 7 Hz) we enter the Theta wavelength, the half-asleep or dreaming state. When we are in deep and dreamless sleep our brainwaves have slowed down to between 0.5 and 4 Hz, which is the Delta range.

THE ALPHA STATE

Generally speaking, being in Alpha is more blissful than being in Beta, unless you get 'high' on excitement, danger or

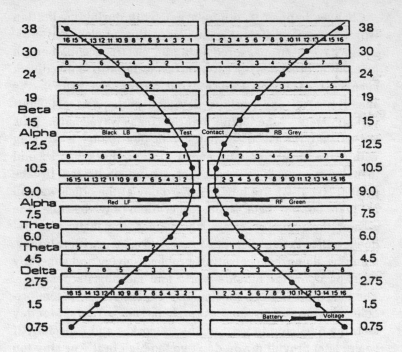

Figure 1A: Beta States

the challenges of your work. But you cannot live on adrenalin all the time, and when you do decide to ease off, the euphoria of Alpha is experienced even more, in relaxation or celebration of the success of your efforts. Alpha is the most *pleasant* state of awareness to be in. It has in fact been likened to being awake, yet in a sleeping body. In other words, a combination of a calm, clear, tension-free mind and a body that is totally relaxed. It is this Alpha state that is facilitated by meditation and which we sometimes refer to as the 'meditative space'. And it is in this Alpha space that tension evaporates, batteries get recharged, the ravages of daily stress are repaired, and we experience a sense of self and of wellbeing, of 'all being right with the world'.

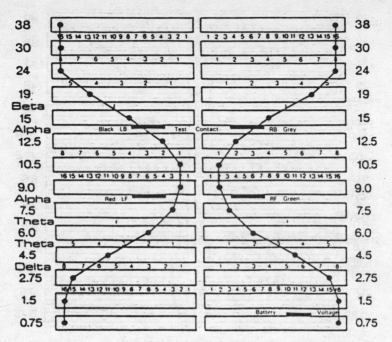

Figure 1B: Beta States

On pages 24–7 you can see what these brainwaves look like when registered on the 'Mind Mirror', a biofeedback machine invented by C. Maxwell Cade and an engineer named Geoffrey Blundell. The Mind Mirror is a portable two-channel machine which analyses signals from both hemispheres of the brain and registers them on a monitor screen as little red lights. The prototype was used first by Maxwell Cade on one of his courses in meditation and relaxation in June 1976, and the perfected model is still being used today on similar courses run in London by his widow, Isabel.

Connecting up with the Mind Mirror, one can see when one is functioning predominantly on the Beta wavelength and when one is moving down into predominantly Alpha

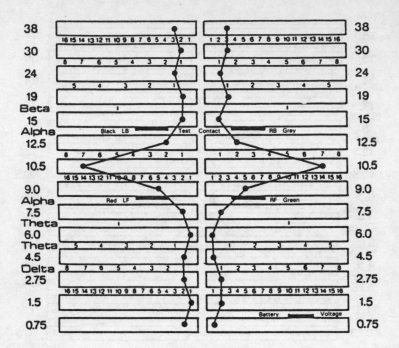

Figure 2A: Alpha States

frequencies, feel what one is experiencing subjectively while this shift is happening – and learn how to facilitate the process in order to be more relaxed. (Isabel Maxwell Cade told me recently that many cancer patients are coming to her courses and individual sessions to learn how to achieve the Alpha state that is healing for anyone with an impaired immune system.)

All the lights line up at the centre of the display on the monitor screen when there is no signal. In the diagrams reproduced here one can see the different brainwave patterns that go with different states of mind, feeling and movement. The numbers down the outside of the diagrams show the

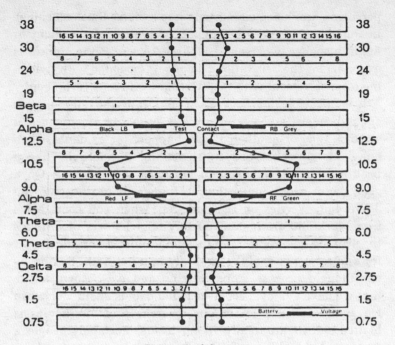

Figure 2B: Alpha States

frequency, ranging from 38 Hz (Beta) to 0.75 (Delta). The small numbers along the horizontal lines indicate the amplitude of the signal (the 1–16 figures are measured in millionths of a volt). Movement towards the left of the red light shows the degree of left hemisphere activity, and movement to the right of right hemisphere activity. It will be seen that, as well as Beta and Alpha waves, there are other frequencies present, but not as predominantly.

Figures 1A and B show typical Beta states of a subject still mainly preoccupied with things going on in the world outside, thinking a lot and experiencing some tension (which could be associated with the normal unsureness of the average person on first being connected up to a biofeedback machine). In Figure 1B we see the high Beta typical of the 'fight or flight' response, whereas in Figures 2A and B the subject is experiencing the 'relaxation response' associated with switching off involvement with the external world and 'turning in'.

It is possible, of course, to slip into the Alpha state spontaneously, and everybody has probably experienced it at some time or another. It can happen, for example, when one is totally absorbed in something pleasurable, like a beautiful sunset, listening to music or making love. On a good day it may happen that, in the words of the song, you 'leave your worries on the doorstep' when you come home from work and are instantly ready for whatever nice things the evening has to offer. Luxuriating under a shower does it for a lot of us, or soaking drowsily in a hot bath. By and by our thought process stops buzzing and we become aware that we have a body, become *sensual* beings again. For when we are thinking, a lot of our awareness of our bodies is blotted out: we are totally 'in our heads'. For many people, a favourite hobby like gardening, for example, does it for them, as indeed does contact with nature generally. All these activities can be meditations if their effect on us is to bring us out of Beta into Alpha. Anything can be a meditation, depending on how totally we absorb ourselves in it, 'lose our minds' and 'come to our senses' – even stroking the cat. Dr Aaron Katche of Pennsylvania University found that petting an animal to which one is bonded leads to lower blood pressure. He discovered that, of 932 coronary patients between 1975 and 1977 followed up one year after discharge from hospital, only three of the fifty-three pet owners had died compared to eleven of the thirty-nine without pets. It is not surprising that the cat has always been considered as having things to teach us about total relaxation. Observing my own cats, they seem to spend most of their day in something that looks suspiciously like the Alpha state. If I wish to pet them but am still high in Beta – tense, speedy and perhaps too abrupt in my movements – and do not tune into their relaxed sensuality they will simply take themselves off in search of more relaxed vibrations elsewhere.

We *can* get out of Beta and into the Alpha state otherwise than by formal meditation. But it is a hit-and-miss affair. Sometimes our minds simply will not switch themselves off. And the more we have used them during the working day, the more likely they are to want to go on running when we would rather switch off.

To meditate regularly is deliberately to structure within our day a time for treating ourselves to the experience of the Alpha state, with all the benefits that this brings. As we have suggested, these benefits include not only relief from mind pressures and emotional clarity and tranquillity but also a recharging of our batteries and balancing of our bodily energies that is healing at a very deep level. 'An Alpha a day' really does help to keep the doctor away.

2
PATHWAYS TO ALPHA

Sitting quietly,
Doing nothing,
Spring comes and
The grass grows
By itself.

Zen *haiku*

It was in the search for wholeness and spiritual enlightenment that meditation evolved first in the East. Those who reflected most deeply on the human condition came to the same conclusion: that our deepest problem is that we are not masters in our own homes. Long before the modern discovery of the Unconscious and its ability to sabotage our best intentions – or, indeed, of St Paul's famous *cri de coeur*: 'For the good I would I do not; but the evil which I would not, that I do' – eastern thinkers were aware of a basic split in the human psyche between the urge to *be* and the urge to *do*. For the Taoists, this compulsive doing takes us away from experiencing 'just being', our oneness with the Tao – with Nature, with Life – which alone can bring inner peace. To get caught up in the 'Ten Thousand Things' (the world of doing) is a dead end: all we will get for our efforts is suffering, frustration, exhaustion. So the Taoist sage Lao-Tzu tells us that 'Stillness and Tranquillity set things in order in the Universe' and advises us to 'practise non-action, work without doing' (*Tao Te Ching*, chs 45, 63).

The mark of the Sage (i.e. an enlightened or self-realized person) is effortlessness. It is not that he actually does nothing, but that he is not a compulsive doer, and when he does act it is a necessary response to the situation, no more, no less. The only discipline of the Taoist is to 'abide in the Tao' – to stay flowing with what is, adapting himself to changing conditions, just as water adapts itself to the container it happens to be in.

In the Bible this Taoist state of primordial at-one-ness with Life is represented by the Garden of Eden, in which our first parents enjoyed 'just being' in the same way (one assumes) as the plants and the animals. Until, that is, Adam and Eve allowed themselves to be seduced by mind (the Serpent) into eating of the Tree of Knowledge, thus starting a whole new ball game that we have had to play willy-nilly since, namely, feeling exiled, out in the cold and trying desperately to get back home again, rather like poor ET. But an angel with a flaming sword stands East of Eden preventing us from going back – appropriately, for a sword is a symbol of mind's capacity for discrimination and analysis, and it is precisely this that splits us off from experiencing our primal innocence and oneness with Creation. We should rephrase Descartes' dictum 'I think, therefore I am' to read rather, 'I think, therefore I do not experience who I am'.

It is only recently that we have learned to understand why this is so, with the discovery of the different functions of the two hemispheres of the brain. Thinking is a function of the left side of the brain, while feeling – which is what experiencing basically is – is a function of the right side of the brain. This is why, if we want to feel more, we have to think less. We have to 'lose our minds' and 'come to our senses' – the domain of the right brain hemisphere. But we have become so addicted to thinking that often we confuse this with feeling. It is a common experience, for example, to ask someone what they are feeling and to be told what they are *thinking* – albeit prefaced by the words 'I feel'. This is similar to the usual answer to a request for information about who someone is: more likely than not you will be told what they do for a living. Thinking and doing are really aspects of the same left-side brain activity, for thinking is internalized doing. Our educational system (with a few notable exceptions) rewarded us for being good at both and did not show much interest in how we were *feeling* as, day in, day out, we sharpened the mind sword and learned the 'doing' skills that would enable us to earn our living and contribute to society. An indispensable part of our 'doing' and 'thinking' activities is the identification of symbols by which we try to impose a sense of order on what we feel – on our immediate experiences of 'being'. Using symbols in this way is a convenient form of shorthand – we do not have to describe the concept or the image each time. This is fine so long as we do not forget that the symbol is not the reality. In the process of 'doing' rather than 'being', we have become so proficient in using symbols to represent reality that we confuse the two, and think that by labelling a thing we therefore *know* it, truly experience its 'isness'. The danger in this is that we may pull the wings off the butterfly in our zeal to understand it. The menu is not the meal, the map is not the territory.

Alpha is very much a right-side brain phenomenon. In other words, it comes to us when we move out of the functions that are the speciality of the left brain hemisphere – thinking, analysing, doing, verbalizing – into the world of the right hemisphere, the world of sensing, intuiting and feeling. Meditation – the high road to Alpha – is therefore, not surprisingly, very much about the *recovery of feeling*, the capacity to experience the world directly, to *know it* without the intervening filter of ideation and labelling that passes for knowledge. I say 'recovery' of feeling and direct experience because we had it as children, but have since been educated out of it.

In a sense, therefore, meditation is a de-conditioning, a

breaking of habits of compulsive thinking. To meditate is to restore the balance of the brain's two hemispheres.

But the mind does not switch itself off that easily. It is almost as if it fights for survival. It will bombard us with thoughts – any thoughts – rather than stay with no thoughts at all, which would feel like death to it. So 'switching off the mind' is something we ourselves have to learn to do – and expect to be resisted all the way.

An enlightened person is one who has 'dropped' the mind. In other words, is not controlled, manipulated or brought down by it, can use it for its proper functions, and put it on one side when it is not needed. Unlike most of us, he does not believe everything he tells himself – and even less, act on it. Eventually the mind is brought to heel, and follows its master obediently like a well-trained dog, rather than dragging him wherever it wants to go. Yes, it is possible, but nobody said it was easy. And yet the attainment of what in zen is called 'No Mind' is such a blessing and a boon that countless people throughout the ages (and today) are prepared to work hard, experience discomfort and self-sacrifice in order to obtain this 'pearl of great price' which we may call 'peace of mind'.

Masters throughout the ages have given their disciples clues as to how to bring the mind to heel. Based on their own experience of what worked for them, each emphasizes a different approach. But these meditation techniques have much in common. First, none of them seeks to tackle the mind directly, because to fight it is to make it stronger. In fact, one part of the mind would be fighting another, so we would split ourselves even more. Rather than resisting thoughts, we allow them and watch them come and go. This 'just watching', or 'witnessing', is the most passive activity a human being can engage in. It is the opposite of 'doing'. Another thing all meditation techniques have in common, and a corollary to this passivity, is that they seek to trick the mind into slowing down. As the treadmill slows down it is easier to get off it. Gaps in the procession of thoughts appear, like patches of blue sky behind clouds, and through these gaps we slip into the peace of the Alpha state more easily. And, whatever the meditative approach, the end-product is the same. In 1961 in New Delhi Dr B. K. Anand found the same increases in Alpha brainwave activity in yoga practitioners as were discovered five years later in zen meditators by Drs Kamasatsu and Hirai of Tokyo University.

So what are these 'pathways' that have been found to work in bringing us out of our everyday mind with all its turmoil and tension to the blissful experience of at-one-ment, Alpha, 'peace of mind' – call it what you will? We list them below, and in Chapter 3 we describe some techniques of meditation which incorporate them.

WITNESSING

The essence of any form of meditation is giving passive, relaxed attention. This is not the same as concentration. Witnessing is more an open-ended state of awareness, an 'expanding to include' and a 'staying in touch' at a feeling level with whatever is being witnessed. Concentration is a left-side brain phenomenon, penetrating the object of concentration for a purpose, usually to understand it better or to see it more clearly. Witnessing, on the other hand, is less 'male' and more 'female', allowing the object being witnessed to be there just the way it is, and feeling it. Concentration seeks to grasp and to control, whereas witnessing allows us to be taken over by what is being witnessed. It is the difference between racking our brains to remember the name of the rose, and simply allowing ourselves to enjoy its colour and fragrance.

At the same time as giving relaxed, unjudging attention to the object being witnessed, we are also aware of ourselves as the witness, as if the point from which we are witnessing is midway between, say, ourselves and the rose. The effect of this is to expand our consciousness by 'taking us out of ourselves', counteracting the tension and contraction of awareness that goes with being preoccupied with our problems.

In Buddhist meditations like *vipassana* (page 74) the meditator simply sits and witnesses his or her own thought process without getting involved in thinking. Thoughts will come: worries will surface and seek to drag us into worrying; memories will try to lure us into reminiscing about the past; thoughts about our commitments and programmes will entice us into thinking about the future and all the things we have to do. But the meditator 'sits fast', like the Watcher on the Hill, observing the comings and goings in a detached and aloof way. With luck. For, at least in the beginning, until you get the knack (which is all meditation is), you will lose the witness space time after time as a particular thought manages to seduce you out of it – and you find some minutes later that you have got lost in pursuing a particular line of thought. So then you have to return to witnessing over and over again, without blaming yourself – or rather, including in your witnessing the part of you that is impatient with your lapse of awareness and detachment.

Meditation does become easier with practice. Remember that to meditate is to break a lifetime's habit of being dragged wherever your thoughts take you. Meditation is like training an animal: it takes time, patience and gentleness before the beast gets the message that it now has a master and can no longer do just anything it wants. In zen there is a famous series of pictures representing symbolically the process of bringing the mind under control (see pages 37–8). The mind is portrayed as an ox, used to running wild and doing as it will. We first see the tracks of the beast when we begin to suspect that the remedy for our restlessness and malaise must be sought within ourselves rather than repeatedly trying to change our outer circumstances. As we start to look within in meditation we see the ox more clearly – the nature of mind and its unruliness. The rest of the ten pictures depict the taming of the animal and the subjective state of oneness and peace that go with it. Another eastern model sees the mind as a monkey, leaping randomly from branch to branch, never still, gibbering endlessly. And indeed, the more one meditates, the more one comes to realize how much of what we tell ourselves inside our heads is pure gibberish.

For a beginner, to try witnessing meditations like *vipassana* and *zazen* is like jumping in at the deep end. They are the hardest to stay with, simply because the rewards – stillness, peace, bliss – come only with a dogged persistence that refuses to be put off by initial boredom, discomfort and definitely wanting to be anywhere else except sitting on a cushion being tormented by one's mind. For this reason, even though they are what most people think of as 'meditation', we give them last in the meditation techniques in Chapter 3.

ONE-POINTEDNESS

As we have said, to tackle the mind 'head-on' by trying to stop the thought process does not work. We will only make ourselves more tense by resistance and strengthen the mind, which will now control us in the form of the thought 'I must stop thinking'. Instead, we have to seduce the mind into slowing down. We do this by giving it something to occupy it, so that at least the monkey stops leaping about all over the place and stays on one branch. In meditation, this is called 'one-pointedness'. This does not mean *concentrating*, but rather centring one's awareness and giving passive attention to one thing at a time, rather than being scattered, distracted by thoughts of this, that and the other. Since the Beta wavelength is very much about being preoccupied with the 'Ten Thousand Things' (e.g. those letters I have to write;

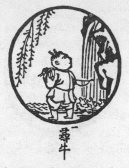

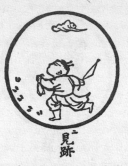

1. It begins to dawn on me that my mind is a distorting mirror and that things are not always as they seem.

2. As I become more aware of my own mind I become more aware of the projections and interpretations of others.

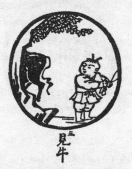

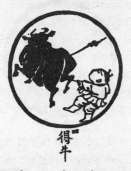

3. Starting to meditate, I begin to realize the extent of my conditioning.

4. Restless, mind wandering, I try to witness my thought process.

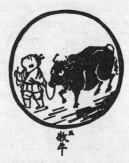

5. Little by little, as I meditate, gaps appear between thoughts.

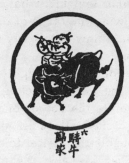

歸騎六
眾牛

6. I am no longer driven by my
thought process.

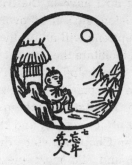

忘七
牛人

7. Serenity at last! The restless
chattering has stopped.

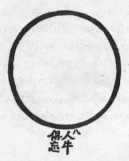

人八
忘牛
俱

8. No-mind is here to stay.
The mind is now my servant.

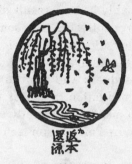

返九
還本
源流

9. With no barrier of mind, I now
experience the world directly, in
all its colour and freshness.

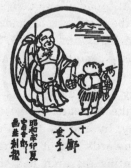

入十
鄽
垂
手

10. When I am enlightened, I see
everybody as enlightened.

what do I have in the fridge for dinner tonight?; what's on television, etc.), it follows that narrowing the range of one's perceptions will naturally slow down brainwave activity and thus facilitate the descent into Alpha.

It also helps the shift from left-side brain to right-side brain to 'come to one's senses', into the world of feeling. So many meditation techniques incorporate the use of one or more of our senses, and these types of meditations are given first in Chapter 3 since they are probably the easiest to stay with and the most pleasurable. They are also the most familiar to us, since if we do happen to slip spontaneously into the Alpha state in the course of our normal day, it will probably be as a result of one or other of our senses having been captivated by something (e.g. beautiful flowers, a garden, a painting, music, making love), temporarily blotting out the mind's activity and giving us the experience of one-pointedness and total absorption – which is another name for meditation. Some of the ways in which you may have been meditating already without knowing it are in fact time-honoured meditation techniques.

LISTENING

It is a common experience that the more disturbed we are, the less we listen. Often, in arguments, we are so caught up with rehearsing what broadside to deliver next that we don't actually hear what the other person has just said. If we have a resistance to hearing what we don't want to hear, we won't. We are 'closed', contracted, tense because we feel threatened.

To listen properly opens us up. It is an allowing in, and therefore passive, like the ears. And if we are listening to, say, music we enjoy, by and by the mind slows down and energy moves downwards out of the head into the body – and we relax. Scientific research has shown that all living things respond to music. (Interestingly, while plants flourish on Vivaldi, their growth is either stunted or abnormally accelerated by being exposed to hard rock.) It has been found in experiments that music increases bodily metabolism, affects respiration, pulse and blood pressure, and changes muscular activity. It is a powerful mood changer: think of what a party is like with or without it, and the different energy it can generate in the audience at, say, a classical concert, a church service or a rock festival. One of the simplest meditations is simply to relax and listen to music – or the sounds of nature (e.g. running water, the ocean, birdsong). It has been found that the best type of music for relaxation purposes is instrumental rather than vocal, and particularly baroque or New Age. As well as facilitating Alpha, baroque music has been found to harmonize the two hemispheres of the brain. Mozart, apparently, is particularly good for co-ordinating breathing, heart and brain rhythms, as well as boosting health generally. (By contrast, Led Zeppelin has been found to inhibit muscle strength!) Some suggestions of tapes to accompany meditations are listed in the Appendix.

Music is not the only form of sound that traditionally has been found helpful as a facilitator of the meditative space. As we have seen, chanting is becoming increasingly popular today as a form of meditation, while mantra meditation in the form of Transcendental Meditation® has been learned by over three million people world-wide since its foundation in 1957. And yet both chanting and holding a mantra as methods of transforming consciousness are much older, and have been used in both Buddhism and Christianity for many centuries. Recitation of the Heart and Diamond Sutras is standard practice in both Hinayana and Mahayana Buddhism (including zen). In the Christian tradition we have not only hymns, but the Rosary and Litanies as well, while in the Orthodox Church a favourite mantra is the 'Jesus Prayer', sometimes called the 'Prayer of the Heart'.

The power of chanting or repeating a mantra to bring us to the Alpha state is no doubt largely to do with the simple fact of repetition having a hypnotic effect, together with the one-pointedness induced by staying with the same formula. But devotees of chanting claim also that the actual formula used is significant and has its own power. Peter Dean, for example, claims that the chant *Nam-Myo-Ho-Renge-Kyo* helps him 'get into the rhythm of life'. Perhaps the most famous chant (also used as a mantra) is *Om*. It is said to be the primal sound from which the whole Universe arises.

Certain sounds are also claimed to have a purifying effect on the energy centres of the body known as chakras, which we shall describe later.

CONTEMPLATION

Contemplation is associated with prayer and devotion in the Christian tradition. And there is no doubt that both of these are effective for very many people in securing blessed moments of peace from the worries and cares of everyday life. Not surprisingly, because, quite apart from religious beliefs, both the trust that goes with praying and the descent of energy from the head to the heart that goes with devotion are powerful antidotes to the ceaseless worrying and worldly preoccupations of the mind that keep us in Beta.

To bring us into a meditative space, contemplation does not necessarily have to be of a devotional nature, i.e. of a religious picture, statue or object. To contemplate is simply to let our eyes rest steadily on some chosen object and to *feel* it – or, as the Buddhists say, to *become* it. Any object will do providing it does not have disturbing associations for us, thereby stimulating the thought process. In Chapter 3, Some Meditation Techniques, we suggest gazing at a flower or a lighted candle, but feel free to select your own object of contemplation.

'Gazing', as it is known in yoga (*tratak*), has to be done in a relaxed, not tense, way, keeping the eyes soft, rather than concentrating. Normally we put out a lot of energy through our eyes, and ceaselessly take in information about our environment through them. By restricting the movement of the eyes to one object we automatically reduce the information being fed to the mind to process, and therefore it has to restrict its prattling to the object being contemplated. Very soon it will run out of things to say and shut up.

Gazing is the exception, together with *zazen* and the 'Third Eye' Meditation (page 137), to the general rule that the eyes are kept closed during meditation, simply to cut out sensory input and to facilitate 'going within'. It has been found with biofeedback that, except in the case of experienced meditators, it is harder to attain the Alpha state with the eyes open than with the eyes closed.

PRESENT-CENTREDNESS

Most meditation techniques are multi-dimensional. That is to say, they work in more ways than one to get us out of Beta into Alpha. Some work with sense withdrawal, some with sense 'expansion-to-include' — it really does not matter, so long as you, not your mind, are in charge. Remember that meditation is a means to an end, a 'knack' for stilling the mind, so you should not get too obsessive about the 'how' of getting into the meditative space. The important thing is to get there, and in later chapters we shall be suggesting ways in which you can make up your own meditation techniques, discovering the knacks that work for you to stay centred in the course of a busy working day, or to 'keep your cool' when everyone around you may be losing theirs.

Like one-pointed awareness, present-centredness is another essential ingredient of every meditation technique. In fact, 'being here now' could be said to be the goal of meditation, for when we are truly in the present moment, experiencing what is, directly through the senses, mind ceases. This is because our minds are like filters between us and direct experience of the present moment, what is going on *now*. Our thought process is concerned with *then* – the future or the past – and our attention can only be in one place at any one time. We are where our attention is, and if it is *there*, *then*, we cannot be *here*, *now*. Our bodies may be (though if we are not aware of them then, existentially, they do not exist, at least in our awareness), but *we* are not. For, re-member, who we really are is not our thoughts but our consciousness, 'the container, not the contained', the *thinker* of thoughts.

Staying in the present moment and allowing ourselves directly to experience and respond to the what is happening *now* at a feeling level (i.e. in right-side brain) rather than out of past habit or *thinking* about it (left-side brain activity) is both a discipline and the goal. Jolting a head-tripping disciple out of thinking into being – and being truly present – is virtually all a zen master does. And the ways in which he does it are sometimes disconcerting for a disciple who is seeking to impress him with clever, intellectual answers to the *koan* (a question which is usually nonsense and quite answerless) given by the master to the disciple in order to exhaust his thinking process to the point where the mind temporarily gives up. The unfortunate disciple can get clouted, have his nose painfully tweaked, or be hit by the master's flying sandal as he flees from the room at the master's roar of disgust. It is a de-conditioning. The student of zen is no longer being rewarded for being clever as he has been trained to be by society. He will earn the master's approval only for being *real*, responding spontaneously and authentically and 'from his gut' rather than from his head.

Present-centredness is about freshness: about de-automatiz-ing ourselves from old repetitive habits of seeing and reacting from habit, practising looking at what is happening around

us with fresh eyes and responding to situations in an un-
mechanical way that combines spontaneity with ap-
propriateness. It is not only in zen that we find masters
insisting on living in the present rather than in the past or
the future. Jesus too urges us to 'become as little children'
(who are so absorbed in the 'now' that they have very little
sense of either the past or the future), to let the dead bury
their dead, not to worry ourselves about the future, for
'sufficient unto the day are the evils thereof'. If we don't, we
miss experiencing the magnificence of the 'lilies of the field'
– which is happening right now.

The pay-offs of 'being here now' include not only relief
from brooding over regrets from the past and worries about
the future but also the increased *aliveness* that comes from
staying closely in touch with changing energy (our own and
that coming at us from the outside), and savouring the
unique flavour of the present moment as intensely as we can.
For what are our lives but the sum total of these moments?
Each moment unlived fully is but an impoverishment of the
quality of those lives.

AWARENESS OF BREATHING

Our breathing patterns and states of mind are very closely
connected. One has only to think of the regular, deep breathing of sleep, the shallow panting of someone who is very
afraid, the suspension of breathing of someone who is deeply
shocked. Specific breathing exercises, designed to raise
energy (*prana*), called *pranayama* are very much a part of the
practice of hatha yoga. But for the purposes of meditation
practice, we are more interested in breathing as a means of
focusing our awareness in the present and on the body.

Becoming and staying aware of one's breathing is one of
the simplest of meditation techniques, and therefore one very
suited to beginners (page 62). Once again, this technique
works to still the mind on several levels. Counting the breaths

(usually after the exhalation) encourages the one-pointedness of our attention. Breathing is very much an ongoing activity in the present moment, so staying with your breathing involves 'being here now'. The regularity of the breathing rhythm has a calming effect and slows down the thought process. If we do lapse in our counting of each breath and fall instead into the trap of following a particular line of thought instead, we realize it immediately, drop the thought and return to counting. Most important, perhaps, is that becoming aware that we breathe at all reminds us that we have a body.

BODY AWARENESS

One of the things that happens when we are busy in the outer world or preoccupied with our thoughts is that we lose awareness of our bodies. All our energy goes into what we are giving attention to, either things or thoughts. It is as if our bodies temporarily cease to exist and we become for the time being just 'talking heads'.

When we sit in meditation and switch off the mind, the energy has to go somewhere, and starts to seep downwards. We start to become aware of body sensations again, of our posture, of the feel of the cushion or chair supporting our buttocks, the position of our hands ... One of the purposes of adopting the type of meditation posture to be described is that it stops energy leaking away. With nowhere to go except in and around the closed body circuit we have made by sitting cross-legged and joining our hands together, energy builds up. We feel recharged, more grounded and centred. With more awareness of our bodies, not only do we feel more alive, but also more relaxed. For body awareness is the *same* as relaxation: it is the 'essential ingredient' in all relaxation techniques, from yoga to autogenics and progressive body relaxation. Relaxing the body helps to relax the mind. It is hard to relax deeply if you are not in a comfortable position

– and easier to 'drop off' and take a nap if you are. Relax the body and the thought process starts to slow down – and vice versa. It works both ways, for in reality body and mind are not separate. We are Bodyminds.

The importance of cultivating body awareness as a pathway to stilling the mind was the great contribution of hatha yoga to the search for enlightenment, which has been described as the ultimate in total relaxation – a letting go of all anxiety and tension and living fully in the moment.

MOVEMENT

How we 'get back into our bodies' again after a hard day at the office varies with all of us. Luxuriating in a hot bath or under the shower does it for some, going for a swim or a jog for others. Without knowing it, we could be meditating when we do these things, moving our energy down from head to body, slowing down our brainwave activity from Beta to Alpha frequencies, 'coming to our senses' again from left-side to right-side brain functioning. Meditation is a very natural process: we may not call it that but we are doing it all the time. But unless we are doing it consciously, as we have said, whether or not we end up in Alpha is a hit or miss affair. To be sure to reap the benefits, it helps if you know what you are doing and to be able to recognize the process while it is happening – otherwise you might miss it. And always, the big question is: is my mind slowing down (while I'm swimming, jogging, etc.) or am I still locked into compulsive thinking? Am I truly *present* here (in this swimming pool, park) right now, or am I (i.e. is my attention) still at the office? Am I *feeling* what I'm doing in this moment of time, or am I *thinking* about it – or worse, something else?

Movement as a meditation is found in both the Sufi and Taoist traditions and is a time-honoured pathway to inner stillness. One thinks of the whirling practised for hours on end by the dervishes; of Sufi dancing (a mixture of devotional singing and movement practised in a group); of Tai-chi, the weird and graceful working through of prescribed movements in slow motion, that, like other martial arts such as karate and aikido, is becoming increasingly popular today. Less well-known, perhaps, are the Gurdjieffians' dance movements, demanding total attention in their complexity to be able to perform them at all, or Subud's *latihan*, allowing the body to move as it will in response to subtle inner promptings of energy. A modern master, Michael Barnett, uses movements along the lines of mandala patterns in order to raise the energy in his groups to the point where mind drops away. The controversial Indian guru Rajneesh devised structured meditations involving movement (often strenuous exertion, as in the Dynamic and Kundalini meditations) to build up energy as a prelude to relaxing totally into the witnessing space.

In view of what has been said about it being easier to still the mind if the body is still, as in sitting meditation, it may seem paradoxical that some forms of movement can still the mind. But there is random, unaware movement, and there is centred, conscious movement – and it is the latter that brings us to the state of one-pointedness, body awareness and present centredness that is the essence of meditation.

Readers who are fond of dancing will no doubt recall the times when they have got 'high' on it, when they experienced their bodies as flowing effortlessly and spontaneously at one with the music, while feeling still at the centre of their consciousness, the 'centre of the cyclone', as if they were just an observer of their body 'doing its own thing'. It is very enjoyable, even blissful, which accounts for the perennial popularity of dancing. This of course is the Alpha state, and the way into it here has been, once again, 'coming to one's senses' – in the case of dancing, to the listening and kinaesthetic senses. But for dancing to be a meditation and not just a 'social shuffle' round the dance-floor it has to be total: we have to give it all we've got, getting lost in it – including our minds. One wonders in passing whether the predilection of disco DJs for playing music so deafeningly loud is something to do with numbing the dancers' minds so that it is impossible for them to think, let alone converse, and thus facilitate 'total dancing'.

CENTRING

To practise meditation is to remind ourselves who we really are. For, if we are not our minds (and if we are able to *observe* our thoughts that means we are separate from them) who, then, are we? Similarly, we cannot be our bodies, or our feelings, for the same reason: we can observe them, so there must be distance between us and them.

Asking oneself repeatedly the question 'Who am I?' is a meditation technique in itself. It is like a zen *koan*, a device which cuts through the intellectualizing and identifications which Gurdjieff called 'the only sin' (i.e. the only barrier to our enlightenment). For, just as we are not our thoughts, our feelings or our bodies, so we also get to realize with this relentless meditation technique that there is nothing else that, *existentially*, we can say we are. At our deepest level we are not our names, or any other of the labels that society has stuck upon us, like 'men', 'women', 'middle class', etc. These are the *positions* we occupy in this lifetime and, not least, inside the body that is our vehicle. We are neither rich nor poor: this is what we *have* or do not have. Neither are we doctors, teachers, plumbers, housewives or civil servants: this is what we *do*, not what we *are*. Ultimately we are left with nothing, or at least nothing we can get our hands on. But then, if we could, it wouldn't be us anyway, simply because, by being able to grasp it at all, it would be the object of our scrutiny and therefore, once again, separate from us.

If you are feeling numb by now, that is very appropriate.

For the question 'Who am I?' is exactly that: mind-numbing. It is like the hand trying to grasp itself. It can't. Eventually, all one is left with with any certainty is that who I am is the one who is asking the question, though *what* this questioner is is ultimately unanswerable. I know that 'I am', but *who* I am, like Life itself, is a mystery. We are like the Tao itself: 'The Tao that can be named is not the eternal Tao' says Lao-Tzu in the opening lines of the *Tao Te Ching*. Buddha always refused to talk about a 'soul' and referred instead to 'empti-ness'. For the Christian mystics 'self-noughting' was a path-way to their most intense experience of 'at-one-ment'. For when we have dropped all our false identifications there is only essence, 'is-ness', and therefore no separation from God, who also 'is of all names free, of all forms void' (Meister Eckhart). Eckhart went as far as to suggest that 'The eye with which God sees me is the same as the eye with which I see God.'

We are emptiness aware of itself, pure consciousness, a nameless subjectivity to which everything else is an object, not only the outer world (including our bodies), but the inner world of thought and feeling as well. And the way to realize this is simply to 'Be still and know that I am God'. In the Hindu tradition the meditator reminds himself constantly 'Thou art That', and resists the temptation to get caught up in false identification by repeating the mantra *neti, neti* ('not this, not this'). One zen master used to do the same thing every morning on waking, with the quirkiness so typical of zen. He would call himself by name and then have a little conversation with himself, warning himself not to forget who he was in the course of the day. 'Yes, master?' 'Take care to stay aware today.' 'Yes, master.' 'Don't allow yourself to be caught up in all the nonsense outside.' 'No, master.'

The 'Who am I' meditation was the basic technique ap-proach of Ramana Maharshi. One of Gurdjieff's devices to jolt his students into heightened self-awareness was the 'Stop' exercise. He would suddenly shout 'STOP!' while they were engaged in whatever they were doing. Immediately they had to freeze in whatever position they might find themselves, and 'go inside' and feel again who they were. This 'self-remembering' Buddha called 'mindfulness'. For the rest of us today, whose priority is perhaps not so much enlightenment as staying sane in a crazy world, reminding ourselves who we really are when we are feeling stressed, oppressed by our problems, and generally taking things too seriously is to return to an even keel – which is what centring is. It is to remember also that 'This Too Shall Pass', and that Life is a mystery to be enjoyed, not a problem to be solved.

SUMMARY
WHAT MEDITATION IS NOT:
concentrating

making an effort

goal-orientated

following *any* line of thought

trying (including trying to get enlightened)

anything that makes us tense.

WHAT MEDITATION IS:
a non-doing

stilling the mind

allowing the shift from Beta brainwaves to Alpha, and from left-
   side hemisphere activity to right-side hemisphere functioning

deep psychophysical relaxation

an alert but relaxed awareness in a sleeping body

being here now

one-pointedness

being in the body, not in the head

'losing one's mind and coming to one's senses'

experiencing directly instead of through the mind filter

centring in the witness space
dropping false identifications
dropping worldly preoccupations and 'coming home' to one's
  innermost core.

Asked 'What is meditation?', Ramana Maharshi replied: 'It is abiding as one's Self without swerving in any way from one's real nature and without feeling one is meditating.'

Meher Baba, the mystic who spoke not a single word between 10 July 1925 and his death at the end of January 1969, conveyed to his disciples through sign language that meditation was 'A path that the individual cuts for himself while trying to get beyond the limitations of the mind'.

For Patanjali, the father of yoga, meditation is 'union of mind and object' (Yoga Sutras, III, 2). When this one-pointed, totally present-centred awareness is accompanied by a relaxation into the body and by effortlessness in action, the meditative space is there.

3
SOME MEDITATION TECHNIQUES

*If you would spend all your time walking, standing,
sitting or lying down, learning to halt the concept-
forming activities of your own mind, you could be
sure of ultimately obtaining your goal.*

Huang-Po

PRELIMINARIES

Regularity and perseverance are important if meditation is gradually to dissolve old habits. As far as possible,
try to meditate at the same time every day. You will have to
find out when the best time is for you, not only from the
point of view of your commitments, but also your energy.
The morning is not a good time for most of us, either because
we have too much energy to sit quietly, have trouble doing
anything at all until we've had our coffee (not a good thing to
drink before meditating anyway if your aim is to slow down),
or because we are in a rush to get to work or the children off
to school. The best time to meditate is before meals rather
than after when most of your energy will be wanting to go
into digestion and you may tend to feel sleepy. My own
experience is that around midday and/or early evening suit
me best. You may find that meditating just before retiring for
the night is not a good idea. It is true that meditation relaxes
us, but it also energizes us and sharpens our awareness,
which is not conducive to dropping off to sleep immediately
one's head hits the pillow.

As well as meditating at the same time each day, it is

preferable to use the same room for each meditation session. The more a space is used for meditation the more peaceful the vibrations become there – and accordingly the easier it is to slip into a meditative space. Think of any meditation centres you may have visited, or indeed any church you may have been to where regular services are held. You feel the peace as soon as you enter. The 'not thinking' of the people who have meditated there, the trust and devotion of those who have prayed there, leave traces. Thoughts are energy, and energy cannot be destroyed. If you think this is fanciful, remember the hotel rooms you have been in, on holiday for example, and how long it took you to 'settle in', to feel at home there. If many people before you have used the room it will have a 'temporary', 'passing through' feel about it. Their thought forms, maybe anxieties and perhaps quarrels will still be there as ghosts until you impose your own vibrations.

You can soften the energy vibrations in a room in several ways. Thoroughly airing it helps and, unless you have some objection to it, burning a stick of incense. (I find the Indian incense rather too sweet and obtrusive and prefer the subtler Japanese variety.) Flowers not only contribute their own gentle beauty and fragrance, but also provide objects for contemplation if you are working with gazing as your meditation. Putting on a tape of soft instrumental music, preferably baroque or New Age, or of 'environmental sounds' (e.g. the ocean, birdsong, the sound of running water) can be an aid to slowing down and 'coming to one's senses' before one starts the meditation session, though you may prefer complete silence while actually meditating. Lighting should be soft and preferably indirect. There is something intrinsically soothing about candles or nightlights, but once again this is a matter of preference.

Cleanliness is important. What we are doing when we meditate is restoring order to internal chaos, returning to our natural state of feeling in harmony after being pulled in all directions by the demands of our daily existence. It helps if our environment reflects order and harmony – and, preferably, is aesthetically pleasing to our eyes – rather than untidy or, even worse, dirty. So, pick up the laundry you left on the floor when you rushed off to work this morning – and run the Hoover over it (the floor, not the laundry) if necessary, so that you do not find yourself later sitting frowning at the bits and pieces on the carpet in front of you instead of sinking deeper and deeper into blissful Alpha. One of the things meditation does is to make you more sensitive to your surroundings.

Above all, arrange things so that you are comfortable. The more comfortable you feel, the easier it will be for you to relax. If you want, take a shower to wash off the grime of the day and freshen up after that journey home in the rush hour. It is better not to soak in a hot bath before your meditation session, as this will probably make you sleepy. If you are really aching for one, rather make enjoying the bath totally your meditation – and skip the session. How to make bath-time a blissful meditative experience is described in Chapter 4.

Wear clothes that are comfortable and non-constricting, and, in winter, warm enough so that you don't get chilled during your session. Shoes should be removed.

If you have had a shattering day – and especially if you have been exposed to very scattered or negative energy – it could be a good idea to clean your aura before settling down to meditate. The aura is the energy field that surrounds each of us, and it can actually be photographed using a technique invented by a Russian electrician named Semyon Kirlian and his wife Valentina. The aura changes in colour and brilliance depending on the state of our energy, whether it is high or low. Kirlian noticed that when he was ill his aura registered as dim and lustreless, while that of his wife, Valentina, who was well, remained bright and clear.

AURA CLEANSING

1. Using the third and fourth fingers of both hands and pressing firmly on the space between the eyebrows (the 'third eye'), trace a line up over the crown of the head down to the back of the neck and then down to the spine as far as you can reach. Still using the same fingers, pick up at the point you left off and continue pressing firmly down the spine (or rather, slightly to each side of it) and down the backs of the legs (simultaneously) to the calves. Shake each foot to kick off surplus energy.

2. Start again at the 'third eye', this time with the third and fourth fingers of the right hand only. Trace firmly a line up and over the scalp and crown of the head, down the back of the neck, along the left shoulder and the front of the left arm. Finish the movement with a sharp 'brush-off'.

3. Repeat the above, this time using the third and fourth fingers of the left hand and tracing a line over the head and down the front of the right arm.

4. Using the third and fourth fingers of both hands, trace the line up from the 'third eye' over the head to a point on the back of the neck between the ears. Here the hands separate, tracing two lines down the neck each side to join together again at the breastbone. Follow the centre line down the front of the body to the pubis. Both hands now simultaneously press firmly down the lines of the outside of the legs, finishing with a 'brush-off' at the ankles.

5. Shake your arms and hands a few times as if getting rid of drops of water, and shake your body also a few times.

It is easier to get down to Alpha if the slowing-down process has already begun before you start to meditate, rather than if you come in through your front door from the world of the 'Ten Thousand Things' and start meditating straightaway. So relax for a while to help yourself 'come down', rather than plunging into your meditation session and expecting immediate benefits. Resist the temptation to have a drink, unless it is water, juice or tea. Alcohol will cloud your clarity, coffee will speed you up.

Tea has traditionally been regarded as the ideal beverage for meditators. There is the story of the first zen patriarch, Bodhidarma, who, impatient with his drowsiness while sitting in zazen, cut off his eyelids and threw them out of the window. Falling on the earth, they took root and grew into the plant that we call 'tea'. Ever since, tea has been helping to refresh meditators and keep them awake without over-stimulating them. You can take this with a pinch of salt (the story, not the tea) as simply pointing up the sometimes ferocious dedication of zen meditators in achieving enlightenment. The old zen masters were the samurai of the meditation world. We are told that in their zeal for their disciples' enlightenment they would cut off the odd finger, or even the odd head. But don't be alarmed. Just choose tea rather than coffee or alcohol and for preference, herb teas such as camomile, rosehip or mint rather than a stirred pot of black Indian tea with milk and sugar.

The slowing-down process prior to starting your meditation session can also be facilitated by cultivating body awareness in some way. Stretching is good, as is taking a few deep breaths. If you know any yoga, relaxing into a few postures before settling down to meditate is ideal.

MEDITATION POSTURES

Whichever posture you choose for meditation, above all make sure that it is comfortable. There are no prizes for torturing yourself. Quite the contrary: meditation is not about asceticism but about deep relaxation. It is something to be enjoyed, and the goal (paradoxically, achieved when we drop any idea of a goal or achieving anything) is the blissful state of Alpha, a by-product of not-trying and not-doing.

Your chosen posture should be one that you can com-

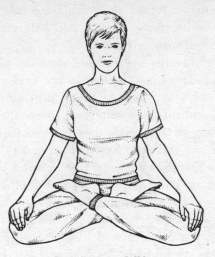

Sitting posture: full lotus

fortably maintain without having to change it for the duration of your meditation session. How long this is is up to you, but in the beginning about twenty minutes will probably feel about right. Arrange not to be disturbed for as long as you intend to meditate, so that you are not jolted out of Alpha back into Beta by having to handle telephone calls or other demands on your attention.

The basic postures for meditation are sitting, kneeling and lying.

SITTING POSTURES

There are several of these, and which one you choose will depend on how supple you are and therefore which feels most comfortable for you. The full lotus posture with feet on both thighs (see above) will probably be quite beyond anyone who does not practise yoga. The half-lotus (page 58) and the 'Perfect Posture' (page 58) are more manageable, the 'Easy Posture' (page 59) even more so. It helps to get and

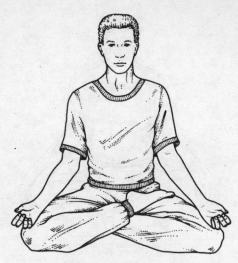

Sitting posture: half-lotus

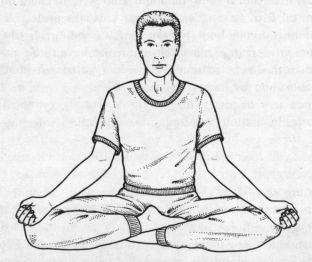

Sitting posture: 'Perfect Posture'

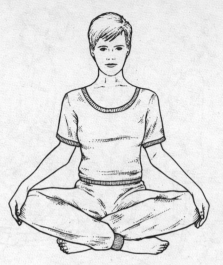

Sitting posture: 'Easy Posture'

maintain the foot on the thigh and both knees on the floor if you put a firm cushion under your buttocks and sit up. If you can keep your knees on the floor it is better, as you will be more grounded. The feeling you should have if the posture is right is that of being securely 'based' on a triangle made by your backside, thighs and knees.

If you can maintain one of these cross-legged postures comfortably without squirming or fidgeting, it is good, because these postures make you feel very grounded and, because you lock yourself into a sort of closed circuit, keep the energy in. But sitting on a chair is almost as good, providing you don't lean against the back of the chair, slouch or cross your legs or feet (page 60). The back should be kept straight (without straining) in all sitting postures. The position of the hands varies, sometimes according to the meditation technique (e.g. zazen), but generally according to your own preference. Thus, the backs of the hands can be resting on the thighs (either palms open or tips of thumbs

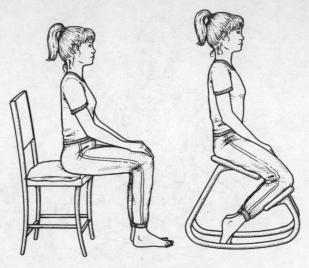

Sitting posture: on a chair

and index fingers lightly touching), or the palms of the hands can rest lightly on the knees, or the hands can be joined in some way, either fingertips lightly touching, or the back of the left hand resting in the palm of the right.

If you are more comfortable sitting on a chair, keep your legs vertical to the floor and do not cross your feet. Above all, once again, keep your back straight without straining. The hand positions are the same as for the cross-legged positions.

KNEELING POSTURE

This will probably be a more comfortable posture to maintain than the cross-legged ones for most people new to meditation. Just kneel, knees together, big toes touching each other, and supporting your buttocks on your heels (page 61). If you wish, you can place a small cushion on the backs of your legs and heels and sit on that. Hand positions, once again, are the same as for the sitting postures.

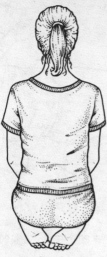

Kneeling posture

LYING POSTURE

Generally speaking, this is not the best posture to adopt for meditation as it is so relaxing that one can easily drop off to sleep, whereas the purpose of meditation is to 'wake us up', in the sense of sharpening our awareness. If, however, you are feeling very drained of energy and are meditating primarily to restore body awareness and recharge your batteries, this 'Corpse' pose (page 62) taken from hatha yoga is deeply relaxing.

Simply lie flat on your back on a carpeted floor or a firm mattress, legs slightly apart. Find a comfortable position for your arms and hands on the floor beside you, palms up.

TIMING

How long you choose to meditate is up to you. Probably more important than the duration of your meditation is its regularity. Try to meditate every day and gradually lengthen the sessions. Initially about twenty minutes should be enough.

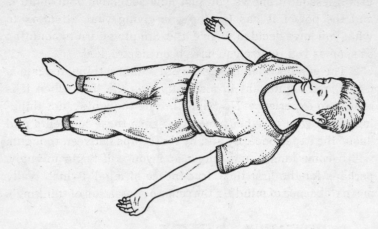

Lying posture: 'Corpse' pose

MEDITATION 1: COUNTING THE BREATHS

TECHNIQUE

This does not involve any special way of breathing, as, for example, in yoga. Just breathe normally, but after each exhalation and before inhaling again count silently 'One' ... (inhale, exhale); 'Two' ... (inhale, exhale); 'Three' ... until you reach 'Ten'. Then start another round with 'One'. Keep your eyes closed for this meditation. As you breathe, feel the air going in and out through the nostrils.

OBSERVATIONS

1. Distractions will certainly come. The most likely thing to happen (perhaps over and over again) is that you will get caught up in following a particular train of thought. The advantage of counting the breaths as a technique is that it is an objective test of your one-pointed attention; for sooner or later you will realize that you have stopped counting. Don't blame yourself, it happens to every meditator and is a

useful lesson: it shows you just how seductive your mind is and the power it has to stop you giving your attention to what you have decided to give it to. Simply return to counting as soon as you realize you have been sidetracked.

2. The gap between breathing out and breathing in again is considered significant in meditation, as the time when it is easiest to experience 'No Mind', i.e. 'no thoughts', 'not thinking'. Be aware of when you experience these moments and 'taste' the experience. By and by these gaps between thoughts will become longer and longer and you will begin to enjoy, perhaps for the first time, true 'peace of mind' (which really means 'absence of mind', in the sense of 'cessation of thinking').

MEDITATION 2: LISTENING

TECHNIQUE
Eyes closed, just listen. This meditation can be done either sitting, kneeling or lying.

OBSERVATIONS
1. What you listen to is not as important as the process of listening. It could be a tape of suitable music or sounds, or simply the sounds coming to you from the outside (e.g. street traffic, a dog barking, the television programme being watched by your children downstairs). The important thing is to be as passive as possible and let the sounds come into you without trying to identify them in any way (or judge them as good or unpleasant, soothing or irritating, etc. – which is typically what the mind will try to do).

2. To help you stay with 'just listening' without evaluating what you are hearing:

try experiencing what you are listening to as a symphony, with each sound adding its own quality, rather like the instruments in an orchestra;

feel what you are feeling as you listen;

become the sounds;

allow any thoughts (probably judgements and associations) to
come up, but don't feed them any attention (either by dwelling
on them or by trying to suppress them) and they will disappear
again.

MEDITATION 3: BEING HERE NOW

TECHNIQUE

Simply sit and let your gaze wander to objects in the room
in turn, observing what is there and really *experiencing*
their reality afresh, as if you were seeing them for the first
time.

OBSERVATIONS

1. This is an exercise in present-centredness and is very
grounding. Usually we have only a rather fuzzy awareness of
our surroundings, especially if they are familiar.

2. Experience each object in turn with as much vividness
as you can – and through your senses. If you like you can
touch and smell the object. Feel the difference between
experiencing things sensually, i.e. feeling them, and thinking
about them.

3. This is a good meditation to do if your mind is particularly active, for example after having to do work demanding a lot of sustained concentration or discussion of ideas.
You will see straightaway the difference between the tension
of concentration and the relief you get from the passive,
sensual awareness of meditation called for here.

4. This meditation gives you practice in directing attention
deliberately to what *you* want to experience, rather than
being pulled out by external stimuli.

5. The one-pointedness required for focusing on different
objects in turn effectively slows down the thinking process.

Your mind will react to your centring your attention probably either with boredom or by trying to think *about*, rather than experiencing wordlessly.

MEDITATION 4: GAZING (*TRATAK*)

TECHNIQUE
Contemplate an object wordlessly, i.e. without talking to yourself about it in your head.

OBSERVATIONS
1. Decide before you start your session what the object of contemplation is going to be. Suitable objects could be a flower or plant, a candle flame, a picture (for example a mandala), but virtually anything will do so long as it does not have negative or disturbing associations for you.

2. Set the object of contemplation on the floor in front of you at a distance that will allow you to gaze at it without straining your neck muscles.

3. Keep your eyes soft. Don't strain or concentrate. You are not trying to look into the object or analyse it in any way. Rather, be receptive to it. Let the attention you give it be as passive as possible, as if inviting the object to come into you. Feel it, become it.

4. When thoughts and opinions about the object try to intrude into your consciousness counteract them by feeling and enjoying the object more.

5. Let your gaze be as steady as possible without forcing. Blink as little as possible.

MEDITATION 5: HOLDING A MANTRA

TECHNIQUE
Repeat silently, again and again, a word or phrase of your choice.

OBSERVATIONS

1. In *The Relaxation Response*, Herbert Benson tells us that experiments have shown that the actual word you choose is not really important, provided, as in the case of the object of contemplation, that it does not have disturbing associations for you. In *How to Meditate* Lawrence LeShan suggests opening the telephone directory at random, selecting the first syllable of each of two names – and joining them together!

2. Some mantras you might like to use are:

Still (or, Stillness)
Peace
Love
Relax
Here-now
Now-here (Nowhere?)

If you are religiously inclined, the devotional associations of the following will also help to still the mind by energizing the heart chakra and thus bring you out of your head:

Jesus
Alleluia
Thy Will be Done

3. As you repeat your mantra, feel which part of your body resonates with it. It will probably be in the heart centre or the lower belly (called in Japanese the *hara* or *tanden*). 'Hold' your mantra in this part of your body, i.e. let your attention focus on this part of your body as you repeat the mantra.

MEDITATION 6: CHANTING

TECHNIQUE

Repeat aloud a specific formula, usually devotional, which is claimed to have the power to energize the body and to transform consciousness. The following are traditional chants that you might like to try (in different meditation sessions) to see which you prefer:

OM (the primordial sound of the universe, pronounced 'home' without the 'h', but, when chanted, more like *AUM* with lengthened vowel sounds)
OM MANI PADME HUM (a chant used by Tibetan Buddhists – literally 'The jewel in the lotus')
NAM YO HO RENGE KO
ALLAH HU (a Sufi invocation of the name of God)
LA ILAHA ILLA' LLAH (another Sufi invocation: 'There is no God but God')
KYRIE ELEISON, CHRISTE ELEISON ('Lord have mercy, Christ have mercy').

OBSERVATIONS

1. Do not intone mechanically, but give each repetition your total attention.

2. Allow your body to resonate with the sound. Become filled with it.

3. After some time, when you have started to make the sounds intensely and to merge with them, you can if you wish change to chanting internally, i.e. soundlessly. 'Intoning' now becomes 'in-tuning'.

MEDITATION 7: BODY AWARENESS

TECHNIQUE

Assume the 'Corpse' pose (page 62) and progressively relax the whole body as follows.

Make yourself very comfortable and take a few deep breaths. Let your awareness move to the big toe of the left foot. Without moving it, let your attention *feel it from the inside*, its size and shape. From there, after a few seconds, let your attention roam over the toes of the left foot in turn. Do not twiddle them; just be as aware of them as you can, one after the other.

Now feel the other parts of the left foot, one after the other. Feel your heel resting on the floor or the mattress, the sole of the foot, the top of the instep, the ankle bone, its hardness, shape and size. Now feel the whole of the left foot. Imagine it as getting heavier and sinking downwards.

Move upwards to the calf of the left leg. Feel how tense or relaxed the calf muscle is. Imagine it expanding, softening, getting heavier. Feel the kneecap, its shape, size, hardness. Do the same for the shin bone. Let your awareness move up to the thigh, front and back, feeling the tension or relaxation there.

Now scan the whole of the left leg and foot. Feel it getting heavier, and notice how much heavier it feels than the right leg and foot. Now 'let go' of your left leg and foot.

Repeat the whole sequence with the other leg, starting with the big toe of your right foot.

When both legs are totally relaxed, allow yourself to become aware in turn of the other parts of your body. Take your time. With each part:

1. feel it first 'from the inside', its size and shape;
2. feel how relaxed or tense it is, and relax into the tension;
3. imagine the part getting heavier, softer, expanding;
4. let go of it.

Feed attention to the other parts of the body in the following order:

buttocks
anus and genitals
lower back
spine
shoulders
left arm: upper arm, elbow, forearm, wrist
left hand: palm, back of hand, thumb, fingers in turn
right arm (as for left)
right hand (as for left)

belly: allow it to soften and 'open up'
chest: breathe deeply into the heart area and exhale with a sigh
   through your mouth.

Now feel the whole weight of your torso. Feel it getting heavier, and your back sinking down through the mattress or the floor. Finish with the face and the scalp, where most of our tension resides as a result of having to 'face the world' and spend so much time 'in our heads'. Allow yourself really to feel this tension before letting go of it. Let your eyes become 'soft', and feel as if they are sinking deep into their sockets. Relax your jaw muscles, letting your mouth sag open. Wiggle your ears to relax the scalp muscles.

By now you should be feeling blissfully relaxed. Enjoy the experience of being totally in your body for as long as you can. If thoughts start to intrude, counteract this by becoming more sensitive to any sensations in your body (e.g. tingles, an itch). You can only give your attention to one thing at a time. Choose not to give it to a thought.

OBSERVATIONS

1. Strictly speaking, this is a relaxation rather than a meditation technique but one ends up in the Alpha state just the same.

2. This technique is perhaps the one you should use to recharge your batteries if you are feeling drained and fatigued and need to bring energy out of your head back into your body as quickly as possible.

3. This is the only meditation technique where it doesn't matter if you drop off to sleep!

MEDITATION 8: *PRARTHANA*

TECHNIQUE

Shoeless, and with loose clothing, lie face downwards. Do not use a pillow. Elbows pointing upwards, place one hand

over the other, palms down, and put them under your forehead so that the knuckle of the index or second finger of
the upper hand presses gently into the 'third eye' space
between the eyebrows. Place the instep of one foot over the
sole of the other. Allow yourself to relax into this posture for
as long as you wish.

OBSERVATIONS

1. This ancient posture is a '*mudra*', a gesture of surrender,
which by its very nature induces deep relaxation almost
immediately.

2. Its relaxing effect – and as a help to avoiding thinking –
can be enhanced by putting on a tape of suitable music
before you assume the posture.

MEDITATION 9: DANCING

TECHNIQUE

Dance expressively and freely, using your whole body and
surrendering totally to the music and the rhythm.

OBSERVATIONS

1. If noise is a consideration, use a Walkman.

2. Wear as few clothes as possible and preferably be barefoot.

3. The music you choose should match your mood of the
moment. Thus, if you have a lot of energy, you could put on some
raunchy hard rock. If you are in gentler mood, try something
more ethereal, perhaps some 'spacy' New Age music that you
can 'float around' to. Whichever you choose, *enjoy* yourself, for
when we are truly enjoying something the mind slows down.

4. You will get more lost in the music and more in touch
with your body if you dance with your eyes closed. Some like
to wear a blindfold. But do be aware of the furniture!

5. Allow your body to move in any way it wants, i.e. in a

way that feels satisfying. Don't try to impose any particular sequence of steps or 'do it right' – nobody is watching you or judging your performance.

6. Dancing becomes meditation when you are totally one with it. It feels as if your body is dancing *you* while you watch, unmoving, from a still point inside you.

7. After dancing, lie down straightaway and allow yourself to feel what you are feeling for as long as you like. If you have put your total energy into the dancing you will almost certainly be feeling good by now, very much in your body, relaxed and not thinking much.

MEDITATION 10: WHIRLING

TECHNIQUE

Whirl on the spot, eyes open but unfocused, right arm held high with palm upwards, left arm low, palm downwards. (Have some cushions strategically placed on the floor nearby so that you can easily subside on to them when you have had enough.)

OBSERVATIONS

1. No food or drink should be taken for at least three hours before whirling. Loose clothing should be worn and feet should be bare.

2. Whirling can be either clockwise or anti-clockwise. Make sure you have plenty of space. Stop straightaway if you experience giddiness or nausea – this technique is not for you.

3. Start the whirling slowly and build up to a flowing movement.

4. As with dancing, the meditation is to experience your body whirling with you as the still centre observing it.

5. At a certain point you will find you cannot remain upright. When this happens, allow your body to subside *gently* on to the cushions. Stretch out immediately into either

the 'Corpse' pose (page 62) or the *Prarthana* posture (see Meditation 8), close your eyes and remain still, feeling what you are feeling, for at least fifteen minutes.

MEDITATION 11: *ZAZEN* (JUST SITTING)

TECHNIQUE
'Sitting quietly, doing nothing . . .'

OBSERVATIONS
1. The eyes are kept half-open in this meditation, unfocused, with the gaze resting at a point on the floor that feels comfortable. You could also sit facing a wall, about six to nine feet away from it, with your eyes lowered so that your gaze rests comfortably. The position of the hands in *zazen* is specific: the left hand is placed over the right, with the thumbs and index finger tips lightly touching, making an 'O'. Just sit. Don't try to do anything – and don't try *not* to do anything either!

2. Particular importance is attached in this meditation to sitting up rather than slouching. In zen monasteries during *sesshins* (meditation retreats involving long periods of *zazen*) one of the jobs of the *roshi* or monk in charge is to spot which of the meditators is dozing off (the shoulders begin to sag) and to wake him up with a couple of whacks on the back with his flat, paddle-shaped stick. (It stings, but is received with gratitude by the meditator. With traditional Japanese politeness, there is an exchange of bows before the meditator resumes sitting with renewed alertness.)

3. Thoughts will undoubtedly come into your mind. If you get caught up in them just come back to observing them as *things* rather than allowing them to lead you by the nose. Kennett-Roshi, a British woman who studied for many years in a zen temple in Japan and now has her own temple at Mt Shasta in California, tells us to watch thoughts as if we were

sitting under a bridge watching traffic going by. Zen master Bassui comments: 'While you are doing *zazen* neither despise nor cherish the thoughts that arise; only search your own mind (or heart) for the very source of these thoughts.'

4. If you feel very distracted, it helps to let your attention focus on the *hara*, the lower part of the belly just below the navel.

5. Don't expect it to be easy and to attain No-Mind straight-away. *Zazen* is an exercise in non-doing. Even if it feels like torture at first you are still learning a valuable lesson about how addicted to doing you are. We all are. Remember that compulsive thinking is *internalized* doing.

MEDITATION 12: ZEN WALKING (*KIN HIN*)

TECHNIQUE

Walk in slow motion round the perimeter of the room in a clockwise direction with intense one-pointed awareness of each step. Walk barefoot or with stockinged feet – no shoes.

OBSERVATIONS

1. *Kin Hin* is used in zen *sesshins* for ten minutes or so in between sessions of *zazen* in order to provide a break from sitting, while yet not losing the meditative space.

2. The hands rest on the chest, one on top of the other, with thumbs intertwined. The back is kept straight as when sitting, but without straining. The eyes remain throughout the walking fixed on the floor a few paces in front.

3. The main focus of awareness should be on the feet and their contact with the floor. Each step is taken with total attention, the heel first making contact with the floor, followed by the sole, then the toes.

4. Zen walking can be done either as a preliminary to *zazen* or as a meditation in itself. It is very centring and calming.

MEDITATION 13: WITNESSING (*VIPASSANA*)

TECHNIQUE

This is similar to *zazen*, detaching yourself from *everything* – thoughts, feelings, body sensations, external impressions – by remaining an impartial observer, the Watcher on the Hill. You simply experience whatever you are experiencing from moment to moment – and *allow* it to be there.

OBSERVATIONS

1. Witnessing is the purest form of meditation there is, and its essence. It is to centre yourself in who you are at your deepest level, which is pure consciousness or pure subjectivity, to which everything else is your object.

2. Become the *container* of whatever you experience by not identifying with the *content*, i.e. the experiences that come and go, like body sensations, thoughts, etc.

3. Stay with *choiceless awareness*. In other words, don't have a preference for pleasant thoughts/feelings rather than uncomfortable ones. (Or if you do find yourself judging and evaluating the contents of your experience, add 'judging' as yet another part of those contents – and watch yourself judging.) Accept with equal passivity and impartiality *anything* that comes – and let it go again.

4. If thoughts and other distractions are particularly troublesome, bring the mind back to one-pointedness by watching the breath coming in and out through the nostrils (as in Meditation 1: Counting the Breaths, page 62).

4
MEDITATION IN ACTION

*The zen master Ikkyu, asked to write some words
of wisdom, picked up his brush and wrote the
word: Attention. The inquirer, puzzled by this,
asked for clarification. Ikkyu then wrote: Attention,
Attention. None the wiser, the questioner
complained that he could see nothing profound in
this. Whereupon, Ikkyu wrote: Attention, Attention,
Attention.*

*A new monk asked the zen master Jyoshu for
instruction in meditation. 'Have you had your
breakfast yet?' inquired Jyoshu. 'Yes, I have,'
answered the monk. 'Then wash out your bowl,'
said Jyoshu.*

If we observe ourselves in action we see just how
often we 'go unconscious'. It is as if while doing something
our minds take us off somewhere else for a while. When we
'come back' we often can't remember where we put things
while we were in these moments of near-somnambulism, for
we have 'lost the thread'. It is as if we fell asleep or went on
to 'automatic' while we were following a train of thought.
Thinking, unless we are thinking deliberately and to some
purpose, is very much like dreaming while awake. We are
where our attention is. We can either be 'in' what we are
doing, or not. Our hands may be making the toast for
breakfast, or in the sink doing the washing up, but *we* may
be far away sunning ourselves on a palm-fringed beach,

perhaps (especially if it is a cold, rainy morning outside the kitchen window), already at the office opening the morning mail, or simply wishing we were back in our warm beds.

What is wrong with this? Nothing, really, provided we are aware that we are choosing not to be here now. We can do what we like, provided we take responsibility and accept what we get as a result. And what we may have to accept if we try to do two things at the same time – the washing up or making toast, *and* daydreaming – could well be cutting our hand on a submerged knife or letting the toast burn. We are just not cut out for doing two things at the same time; it makes for inefficiency and we get the worst of both worlds, or, to change the metaphor, fall between two stools. We don't allow ourselves to enjoy the satisfaction of either relaxing blissfully into a good fantasy or experiencing the zen of washing up or making toast. Being meditative in action means doing one thing at a time, with total attention.

But, I hear you protesting, washing up the dishes is so *boring*. Not, it's not. Nothing is boring, it just *is*. Boredom (and indeed any other experience) is our own creation. Our experience of washing up, like our experience of life, is what we make it, what we bring to it. If we do *anything* out of habit, robot-like, it will always feel boring, stale. And that includes activities that perhaps once got us 'high', 'made us feel' good, blissful, like praying or making love. In reality, nothing can 'make us feel' anything. Our subjective experience is always a function of the quality of attention we are willing to bring to whatever we are engaged in. And the more one-pointed our attention, the fresher, more vivid and intense our experience.

Usually, when the freshness, the aliveness, goes out of things, we tend to move on and try to recapture it elsewhere. We move on from A to B. When B dies on us, we proceed from B to C and so on. A, B, C, etc., could be jobs, lovers, anything in fact. The meditator on the other hand becomes aware that if he or she feels in a rut, it is simply because of not looking. For freshness is always there. Every situation is new, every experience is unique, life never repeats. So, rather than moving from A to B, the meditator works to remove the mind's filter of staleness and habit that imposes a sort of deadness over the activities of daily life. He transforms his experience of A (because A is what is happening right now) by going deeper into it: A1, A2, A3 ... And, unless you can do it with A, you'll never be able to do it with B, C, or D either – 'it' being drinking deep of this experience *now* rather than living superficially, staying always on the surface of things, never really allowing yourself to feel anything at any satisfying level. The mind hankers after excitement, the new, the 'more', which will always be 'out there' somewhere if we can only find it. Meditation, on the other hand, makes us realize that if we cannot be fulfilled, satisfied, contented, peaceful, *now*, we never will. It is to get off the treadmill, to drop our obsession with achieving and acquiring, and to relax into being where we are, and doing what we're doing right *now*, totally.

Try it next time you do the washing up. Instead of doing it with your mind, do it with your senses. Feel the warmth of the water on your hands; smell the fragrance of the dishwashing liquid; watch the iridescent bubbles that try to form on the patches of white foam, and the gleaming knives, forks and spoons as they emerge from it. As you rinse, hear the splashing of running water and feel the stimulating coldness of it after the warmth. Give your attention to making sure every single bit of soap is rinsed off before you stack them, choosing just the right spot for each utensil rather than just slapping it down as it comes.

The point is not the washing up, whether it will be better done for all this; the point is you and your awareness, and bringing your mind under control so that you can give your attention totally to what *you* choose, rather than what *it* chooses. And in the process, you get to enjoy a feeling of satisfaction, of connectedness with the physical world, of inner stillness, that is the result of centring your awareness on one thing at a time, and really feeling and relaxing into what you are doing. As you restrict the mind's activity through your one-pointedness and move over into the right-side brain by 'coming to your senses', by and by you move out of Beta down into the more comfortable, peaceful and satisfying range of Alpha.

Our experience of any activity can be transformed in this way by the quality of the attention we bring to it. Asked 'What is zen?', a master once replied: 'Zen is your everyday life.' Another, asked the same question, answered: 'Nothing special.' In zen monasteries, as much importance is attached to doing the ordinary things of life meditatively as to formal sitting meditation in the *zendo* (meditation hall). Sweeping the floor, fetching water, going to the toilet – every activity is an opportunity to practise present-centredness and giving undivided attention to doing one thing at a time. As Suzuki Roshi told me once in the course of a five-day *sesshin*: 'Everything is *zazen*.'

So practise being more *present* in everything you do in the course of the day. Become more aware, do things more consciously instead of out of habit, robot-like. It is simply a matter of remembering. Your reward will be your increased sense of aliveness, for this is in direct ratio to your attentiveness to the here and now. It is not hard. On the contrary it is as simple as pulling a switch, or waking up. Here are a few examples you could start off with.

WALKING MEDITATION

On the way to the station in the morning to get the train for work, for example, allow yourself to experience the walk *per se*, instead of running over in your head the things you have to do when you get into the office (or wishing you were back in bed!). Let your awareness come back into your body and tune in to where you are and what you are doing, right now. (The Buddhists advise literally reminding yourself of the activity that you are engaged in by repeating to yourself, for example, 'walking, walking'.) Feel, without verbalizing it, what walking is about. It is really quite an amazing phenomenon, how your legs do it without you having to give them instructions every time you place one foot in front of the other. And it is a blessing to be able to walk at all: many people cannot. Watch yourself walking. *Who* walks? What is this witness that can observe walking happening?

Become aware of your surroundings. Don't miss the uniqueness of *this* walk, quite unlike any other you have ever taken to the station before. Expand your awareness to include, perhaps, the beauty of the dawn, or the reflection of last night's rain on the pavement, or the rustle of wind in the leaves of trees that you are passing. Feel the energy of a city beginning to wake up and go about its business, the bustling people, the hum of traffic . . .

EATING MEDITATION

There is a saying in zen: 'Walk or sit – but don't wobble.' In other words, as the old song lyric goes: 'It ain't what you do it's the way that you do it.' Meditation is not about *what* you do, but *how* you do it, whether unconsciously, half-heartedly, or totally and with awareness. So when eating, 'just' eat. Don't read, don't listen to your Walkman, or participate in that heated discussion about politics that may be going on at the table. Do one thing at a time. Eat your food sensually. Chew it thoroughly, experience the different textures of what you are putting into your mouth, the different colours, the different tastes. Even if you don't get enlightened this time round, at least you won't get indigestion.

BATHING MEDITATION

The deeper we go into body awareness, the more blissfully

relaxed we feel. And let us not lose sight of the fact that we are meditating, not in order to 'do it right' or become more virtuous or 'perfect', but in order to feel better than we do. Bliss is the goal, or rather the by-product of meditation.

Make the most of your daily bath or shower. It is a short cut to blissfully 'coming to your senses'. Transform it from a mere cleansing ritual into a deliciously decadent experience. This you can do by:

putting on a tape of suitably soothing, relaxing music that you
　like;
bathing by candlelight: light a candle or nightlight, set it on the
　side of the bath and switch off the overhead light;
make the bath water fragrant with an oil of your preference, e.g.
　rose, sandalwood, lavender.

Now all you have to do is *wallow*. And enjoy. It's the easiest meditation of the lot!

SMOKING MEDITATION

The quickest way to give up smoking is to smoke *totally*. By this I do not mean to smoke more, but to smoke with more awareness. Usually, tobacco addicts smoke while engaged in other things as well: having a drink, chatting with friends, concentrating on work, worrying about household bills. We reach into our pockets or handbag for the packet of cigarettes either through tension or through habit – either way, unconsciously. Making smoking each cigarette of the day an event (which, in fact, it is anyway) breaks the automatism and brings the action of smoking back into the area of deliberate choice – which is the only area where it is possible to say 'No' to it.

So, as for bathing, smoke sensually. Make a ritual out of it. Check whether you really do want a cigarette right now and, if so, *decide* to have one. Feeling the hardness of the packet, note its design and colour (and the health warning!). Open it with awareness, extract the cigarette. Before putting it in your mouth feel its texture ... sniff the tobacco in it. Light up, observing as you do so the colour of the flame of the lighter or the match igniting the tip. Watch the smoke curling up from the end of the cigarette, how it stops when you take a puff, how the tip glows. Experience as fully as you can the smoke coming into your lungs and being expelled again. Feel *exactly* what smoking does for you, what effects you can feel inside your body or in your mood. When you stub out your cigarette, do so deliberately and with total attention. Are you feeling better or worse than you were before you smoked this cigarette?

Friends tell me that giving up the habit is somehow facilitated by highlighting the 'event' of each cigarette even more by noting in a little book you carry around with you the time, the number, and the reason for each cigarette. For our purposes, whether you give up smoking or not is secondary: the important thing, as with everything else, is how mechanical you are. But it is true that the best way to drop a bad habit is not to fight it but to do it with deliberation and awareness each time, i.e. meditatively.

The above are just a few examples of how any of the mundane things we do habitually can be transformed into meditations. Zen has brought this to a fine art in the tea ceremony, in which the whole ritual of making and serving tea is performed with total attention, and in *ikebana*, the art of flower-arranging. In the latter each flower is put in place with a fine awareness of contrast and what looks most natural. This calls for a sensitivity to 'where the flower wants to be' in the arrangement, rather like Castaneda being told by the sorcerer Don Juan to find his 'power place', i.e. the exact spot in a room where he felt 'just right'. Meditation allows us to tune into the world at a feeling level, and thus restores our sense of one-ness with it. This brings with it a grace, a naturalness and flowing quality. It also makes for more efficiency in action, absence of tension and strain. Listening to music, just listen. Jogging in the park, just jog. Swimming, just swim. Do these things totally, don't think as well. *Become* the music, the jogging, the swimming. Merge with it.

EFFORTLESSNESS

In *Zen in the Art of Archery*, Eugen Herrigel describes his training with a master in Japan. Day after day Herrigel practised archery until he was proficient enough to hit the bullseye almost every time. But the master was unimpressed and merely told him to go on practising. As time wore on and still the master would shake his head at what Herrigel considered his faultless technique and, by now, unerring accuracy, the latter got so depressed that he was ready to give up. He prepared to leave for Europe and went to say goodbye to his mentor who had now become more of a tormentor. After they had exchanged ritual goodbyes, the master suggested Herrigel draw his bow just one last time before leaving. Sadly, he did so. He took aim and let go of the arrow. It hit the target, just missing the bull. To Herrigel's amazement, the master let out a roar of approval and came over and slapped him gleefully on the back. 'That's it!' he shouted. 'You got it! Now you can go.'

The explanation of the master's reaction is that, for the first time in Herrigel's long training, the arrow had been shot *effortlessly*. And it had been effortlessness rather than mere technique and accuracy that, from the master's point of view, the training had been about from the very first. Herrigel had been trying too hard, to 'do it right', to impress the master, to hit the bull every time. His ego was very much involved, which meant that, even though he attained proficiency, tension was present in his consciousness, as it always is whenever we are attached to achieving a goal. It was only when he felt a failure and let go of trying that there was no ego, just pure action. The 'doer' had disappeared, and the arrow 'shot itself'.

In the beginning, whenever we are trying to master something new, discipline and effort are needed to acquire the necessary technique or knowledge. Musicians practise their scales, dancers exercise at the barre, aspiring competitive tennis players hit thousands of ground strokes, volleys and services, language students have to be drilled in grammar and correct pronunciation. But once the necessary technique has been acquired through this hard work and has become part of us, we just 'do it'. As Christopher Dean put it after winning an Olympic gold medal: 'It is like a sort of hypnotic trance, in which all the work you have done before comes out of you.' The sign of mastery of anything is this effortlessness, and it is a highly meditative state, combining totally one-pointed attention with relaxing into the activity.

Effortlessness is experienced when you are so much 'into' what you are engaged in that you merge with it. When that happens, you have the experience that there is no 'doer' — that there is only the action being performed as if it were coming through you, but you are only the witness. It is just like when, if you are really enjoying dancing, flowing with the music, allowing your body to move in exact synchronicity with the rhythm, it is impossible to separate the dancer from the dance. There is nothing at all mystical about this phenomenon — which is not to say that it is not intensely satisfying. It happens to us every day when, for example, we get dressed in the morning. We are so used to slipping into our clothes, putting on a tie, tying our shoelaces and so on, we have done this so many times, that we don't have to think about how to do it. It has become a part of us. Regular meditation by and by has the effect of giving us this experience of effortlessness in more and more areas of our lives. As we become more in tune with our inner selves we flow more with what we may be engaged in in the outer world. We become less tense, more spontaneous. Things get easier. Just think of the mess the centipede would get into if he *thought* about every step!

T'AI-CHI CH'UAN

T'ai-chi is included here as an example of meditation in action brought to a fine art. However, it is necessary to find a teacher for this meditation, for the movements are too subtle and complex to learn from a book.

T'ai-chi ch'uan means literally 'supreme ultimate boxing' and is thus one of the martial arts. It is, however, mainly done today as a meditation and enjoys great popularity in China, where people of all ages practise it at dawn and dusk. Its popularity is spreading to the West and occasionally one sees (mainly youngish) people working through the form in our public parks (usually observed with baffled curiosity by passers-by).

It is said that Chang San-feng, a Taoist priest living in the thirteenth century, learned T'ai-chi in a dream. And in fact there is something dream-like about the slow-motion movements that belies the intense alertness with which they have to be performed. The aim is to eliminate all tension in the body so that the *chi* (energy) can flow freely into each movement. It is a training in one-pointedness, present-centredness and effortlessness.

There are several different schools of T'ai-chi and if you are interested in learning it you will find them advertised in health magazines. The traditional T'ai-chi form consists of 128 movements, including repetitions, and takes about fifteen minutes to work through. Some teachers have evolved shorter forms of about forty or fifty movements, taking about ten minutes.

AIKIDO

Aikido is another martial art aimed more at self-development than at self-defence. It was founded over fifty years ago by master Morihei Ueshiba, who had studied many of the traditional Japanese martial arts including judo, ju-jitsu and kendo and was also very much involved in both Buddhism and Shintoism. The secret of aikido, says its founder, is to harmonize ourselves with the movements of the universe and bring ourselves in accord with the universe itself.

It is performed with a partner, but there is no competition. Rather, you practise tuning into your partner's energy, flowing with it, and then seek to redirect it without force, strain or effort. Remaining centred in the *hara* and moving from this vital centre is central to aikido, as indeed it is in other martial arts. Like T'ai-chi, aikido has to be learned with a teacher.

THE ZEN ARTS

Zen has proved extraordinarily fertile in the applied arts. The capacity to give total attention, allied with a totally relaxed body, makes for a fluency in movement and performance that is the hallmark of the meditator.

We have already alluded to Herrigel and the art of archery and seen that the ease and 'let-go' of the archer are considered more important than accuracy. This is true in all the zen arts, where flowing movements and lack of tension is the major consideration. To watch a master doing calligraphy or painting a landscape with deft brush strokes or conducting the tea ceremony, is to witness total present-centredness.

5
MEDITATION, ENERGY AND HEALING

The Body too is a great and necessary principle.
Without it, the task fails and the purpose is not
attained.

Rumi

The concept of energy is central to the holistic
approach to health. Homeopaths and acupuncturists refer to
this energy as *chi*, and illness is considered to be the result
of this energy being too low, unbalanced or blocked in some
way. That human beings are energy fields has been shown in
Kirlian photography (see page 54). Research undertaken in
the USSR and (in the seventies) in the West has demon-
strated that, using Kirlian photography, it is possible to
diagnose certain illnesses before the symptoms become overt.

This symptom manifestation is really the end of a process.
One does not usually 'fall ill', even though it may appear that
way. Disease always starts on finer energy levels as 'dis-ease'
before taking root and manifesting on the grosser, bodily
level. The first sign is usually lowered vitality, vague depression and malaise. Sitting in meditation, tuning in to our
bodies' messages, we can often get 'flashes', i.e. intuit, where
the trouble is building up and why. Perhaps we are not
eating well, or overdoing it at work, or are under some sort
of extra stress. Forewarned is forearmed: if we act early
enough we may well forestall an identifiable illness.

The pioneer of research into stress, Sir Hans Selye, noted
as a medical student how, in the early stages of illness, the
syndrome of 'just being sick' always made its appearance

first: vague aches, upset stomach, feeling unwell and so on. His teachers were not interested in these non-specific symptoms. But, years later, Selye was to suggest that they are significant as registering the body's first alarm signals. More recently, Dr Peter Nixon, consultant in cardiology at London's Charing Cross Hospital, together with Dr David Peters, has been underlining the importance of directing attention to bodily signals when we are in this nether land between being well and not yet having developed specific symptoms of illness. It has been suggested that as many as 70 per cent of the patients who visit their doctor and complain about 'feeling unwell' are suffering from tension caused by stress. In the absence of clear symptoms, however, or something that shows up on an X-ray or in clinical tests, there is very little a doctor can do, apart from prescribing tranquillizers.

We have seen how meditating regularly de-stresses us by inducing a relaxed mind in a relaxed body, and have suggested that 'going down to Alpha' daily is prophylactic against stress disease, the scourge of our time, and that 'An Alpha a day keeps the doctor away'. But we now know that regular meditation also strengthens immunity. What happens when we become stressed is that the hypothalamus in the brain activates the pituitary gland to release hormones that govern the endocrine system. The adrenals go into action and release adrenalin and corticosteroids. Chronically elevated cortisol levels due to unrelieved stress suppress our immune systems. The number of T-helper cells is reduced, while that of T-suppressors is increased. Production of killer cells is inhibited, and interferon (our first line of defence against invading germs) is reduced.

A well-functioning immune system is our biggest single defence against falling ill. Even before the advent of AIDS, much research had been carried out on what strengthens immunity and what wrecks it. In 1976 Gurucharan Singh Lhals, the founder of Boston's Kundalini Research Institute, discovered conclusively that meditating regularly improves immunity. Blood levels of three important immune system hormones went up by as much as 100 per cent. Lhals' findings were confirmed by Alberto Villoldo of San Francisco State College, who in 1980 reported improved white cell response and improved efficiency of hormone response after regular meditation and visualization. It is not surprising therefore that meditation is today being included in health programmes for those whose immune systems are seriously impaired, for example, people with cancer and AIDS.

More recently, one of the interesting facts to emerge from research is the damage that can be done to our immune systems by holding on to habitual negative mental patterns — long-standing resentments, for example, or guilt. These acid thoughts release toxic chemical messengers into the blood, and poison it as surely as they poison our minds. Habitual anxiety, too, feeling unsafe in the world, results in our being permanently geared for fight or flight, and an immune system constantly kept on 'red alert' can eventually become exhausted. The most damaging negativity of all, however, has been found to be that which we direct against ourselves as the result of a too low self-image. It would appear that the biggest single safeguard of our health is to love and accept ourselves unconditionally, and to nourish ourselves at all levels.

Love heals, as does forgiveness, and thinking loving thoughts. It seems that even just dwelling on past experiences of loving and being loved is healing, according to Harvard psychologist Dr David McClelland, who found that 'meditating on love' raised immunoglobulin levels. In research done with his colleague Carol Kirshnit in 1982, McClelland discovered that even watching romantic movies increased levels of immunoglobulin-A in the saliva, our first line of defence against colds and other viral diseases.

The new science of psychoimmunology is proving beyond

any doubt that our mental pictures produce corresponding changes in body chemistry, for better or for worse, for health or for sickness. Miracles of healing can happen, even from 'incurable' illnesses like cancer and AIDS, when negative mental patterns are deliberately replaced by positive images (visualizations) of health and healing, love and forgiveness. The success of Dr Carl Simonton's pioneering work with cancer patients in the USA has led to his techniques being adopted elsewhere, for example at the Bristol Cancer Help Centre and other centres in Britain. Most recently, the British National Health Service has been showing an interest in making these techniques available in public hospitals as a supplement to more orthodox medical treatment. Readers interested in learning more about visualization and other approaches to healing the body through the mind will find the following books interesting and useful:

Getting Well Again by Carl and Stephanie Simonton (Bantam, 1986)
The Bristol Programme by Penny Brohn (Century, 1987)
Loving Medicine by Dr Rosy Thomson (Gateway, 1989)
Self-Healing: How to Use Your Mind to Heal Your Body by Louis Proto (Piatkus, 1990).

MEDITATION 14: *METTA* (LOVING KINDNESS)

TECHNIQUE
Directing loving thoughts to yourself and others.

Imagine that you are breathing out all tension, worry and negativity and breathing in patience, kindness and forgiveness. After a few moments of this, visualize yourself as breathing in either white or pink light. Feel this light permeating your entire body, warming and cleansing you ... Experience yourself as a valuable being, magnificent and special, and send yourself love.

Now see this light extending out from your body to envelop other people, who are just as valuable, magnificent and special. The light is the energy carried by your good wishes for them, your 'wishing them well'. Extend it first to those you love and who you know love you, such as your family and friends. Take your time and try to get a clear picture of each person as you direct this loving energy to them. If you cannot visualize them clearly, just have the intention to nourish them with your love. It will reach anyway.

Now choose to include in your 'kindly light' those you are not so keen on (or even positively dislike, perhaps because they have behaved badly to you in the past). Choose to forgive them and to wish them well. If you feel resistance to doing this, tell yourself that you are not condoning what they may have done, but acknowledging that they are fellow travellers on this planet of ours, made of the same stuff as you, pure consciousness, and therefore as divine as you are. By choosing to love them you are also choosing to love yourself. Don't suppress your resistance, just allow it also to be there – and love yourself for not being as perfect as you would like to be.

Now let your 'wishing well' extend to the whole world, all the people out there whom you do not and will never know. Like you they feel, struggle, make mistakes and generally are trying to do the best they can given their conditioning and circumstances. Let your compassion go out to all who are suffering in any way, from poverty and hunger, ill-health, oppression and injustice, loss . . .

See the earth as if you were out in space, as the astronauts see it, serene, green and beautiful. Wish for it more peace, tolerance and mutual understanding between people. Extend too your compassion to the animal and plant kingdoms that are in pain from our continued exploitation of them.

Finish by coming back to yourself and wishing all these good things also for yourself. You deserve them.

OBSERVATIONS

1. This beautiful Buddhist meditation is not just a pious exercise but psychologically integrating and calming. The loving energy you are encouraging will move energy down from the head into the heart chakra, from thinking into feeling. Also, with the expansion of consciousness, the contraction caused by tension will be dissolved. Directing loving energy towards yourself is also one of the most healing things you can do.

2. Be sure to ground yourself again after practising this meditation (and indeed all meditations of the visualizing type) before you get up and doing again. Open your eyes, look round the room at objects and remind yourself where you are. Clench and unclench your hands a few times and rub them together. Become aware of body sensations.

Metta is an example of 'meditating on the opposite' to transform negativity into positive energy by deliberately focusing on the latter and withdrawing energy from the former. It will leave you feeling calmer and better about your relationships. The following visualization will be useful for counteracting any negative images you may have about yourself.

MEDITATION 15: YOUR PERFECT SELF

TECHNIQUE

Dwelling on your innate magnificence and lovability.

Imagine a being standing in front of you a few feet away. Visualize this being as possessing all the ideal qualities you can think of, as perfect as you yourself would like to be. Whatever are your highest values, ascribe to this being: beauty, honesty, courage, humour, grace, awareness, compassion. Keep going through the list of ideal attributes until you can think of no more. The more positive energy you see in this being, the more radiant it becomes.

Contemplate this radiant and perfect (and perfectly healthy) being, and know that it is your own potential. All these qualities must already exist in you otherwise you would not be able to recognize them. This high being knows this, and as you contemplate him or her silently, blissfully, you hear the words: *I am you and you are me.*

Your perfect being now moves slowly closer to you, closer and closer until you merge with each other. Now there is only *you.* Feel what it is like to be perfect, whole, complete, and feeling a lot of love for yourself. Enjoy this feeling for as long as you wish – and recall it whenever you start to feel bad about yourself again.

Later we shall be suggesting other ways in which the creative power of the mind can be harnessed for dissolving negative patterns of thinking. Here in the meantime are some visualizations to assist your body to make itself well again if you are ill, or to feel better if you are in pain. They are taken from my book *Self-Healing*, where you will find more about using the power of the mind to heal the body. Remember that the body cannot distinguish between 'real' reality and imagined reality. It will obligingly come up with the physical response to match *any* pictures you are projecting on your mind-computer.

MEDITATION 16: VISUALIZING HEALTH

TECHNIQUE
Dwelling on health (as opposed to worrying about how ill you may be).

Conjure up a picture of yourself in perfect health, perhaps as you were before you became ill, or as you would like to feel right now. Imagine yourself well again, with lots of energy, ravenous appetite and feeling good. See yourself in as much detail as possible, enjoying again the activities you used to. Get this feeling in your body.

Keep these images up your sleeve to trot out at the times when you are feeling down and depressed about your health, to counteract the mind which may be telling you that you will never feel well again. Return to this picture of yourself as vibrantly healthy as often as you wish. We grow into what we habitually think about, and create more of it in our lives. So do not return to picturing yourself as ill again – ever.

MEDITATION 17: HEALING A PART

TECHNIQUE

Directing positive healing energy to any part of your body that particularly needs it.

Let your attention focus on the part of your body that is in trouble. It could be a broken limb, an inflamed joint, a wound, or some internal organ that is affected. Relax as much as you can and really try to feel the part that is in distress. What images of it come to mind? Stay with these mental pictures for a while until one seems to be the clearest, most dominant or persistent image – and work with that one.

Start to direct loving attention and intention to heal to what you can see in your mind's eye. The medium for this healing energy you are directing should be such that it cleanses, clears up, soothes, conquers or restores order and symmetry to what you are probably seeing as in some way dirty, dark, disorganized, unharmonious, jagged or otherwise in a sorry state. The agent of healing could thus be a jet of clear, crystalline water, a paintbrush, a mop or a vacuum cleaner – anything in fact that has the power to make clean, purify, restore order, smooth rough edges or clear up a mess.

Persevere with your healing 'restoration work' until it feels finished and the part looks in much better shape than when you started. Remind yourself if your faith in what you are doing falters that, at the very least, you are sending more blood with reinforcements to the part simply by feeding it attention. Try to stay relaxed – don't force it. (Experiments have shown that one can warm one's hands by focusing attention on them – but not if one concentrates too fiercely.)

Here are a few examples, but it is better if you use images that occur to you spontaneously. Adapt the technique to whatever symptom you may be suffering from.

Arthritis. Picture the joint surfaces as pitted. See yourself rubbing them with some soothing but powerful agent until they are smooth again. (This visualization was successfully used by the Simontons' first 'cure', an elderly man who had already used visualization to heal himself of throat cancer.)

Fractures. See the break, and mend it with whatever materials you need, just as if you are repairing anything else that had broken or split, e.g. with glue, Sellotape, etc. Before you leave it, test that it will hold together and leave it to set.

MEDITATION 18: WHITE LIGHT

TECHNIQUE

Visualizing white light penetrating your whole body. Use this for healing generally.

Imagine that you are surrounded by white light. Keep giving attention to this light so that it becomes clearer and clearer, more and more brilliant. Allow this light to penetrate you, entering you through the crown of the head and washing away all toxins and impurities in your whole body. Surrender to this light. Feel it flushing out every nook and cranny, cleansing and energizing. Really try to feel it flowing through you and out through the soles of your feet.

When you feel totally cleaned out, relax for a while and enjoy the sensations of aliveness in your whole body before grounding yourself again.

HANDLING PAIN

Much of what we call 'pain' is in fact tension caused by

anxiety and muscle contraction. Assuming that your doctor has already treated the source of the pain with appropriate medication and has done all that he can do, the only thing you can now do is to try to relax as deeply as you can. The following meditative techniques might help.

BREATHING INTO THE PAIN

Imagine that you are directing healing, soothing energy in the form of white light into the part of your body that is hurting.

DIALOGUING THE PAIN

Ask it why it is there, what message it has for you, and what you can do to ease it.

TRY TO FEEL THE PAIN MORE

Try to relax *into* it. In so doing you will take the edge off it and expand to include it, rather than contracting to avoid it.

VISUALIZE THE PAIN

Visualize the pain as if it were a *thing*. How big is it? What colour? What area does it occupy exactly? What shape is it? As you watch it, the pain will fluctuate in size, shape, colour and the area it occupies. Stay with it, observing and feeling it as much as you can. Often what happens (particularly with tension headaches, though not, alas, with toothache) is that it starts to shrink, to get fainter in outline, less virulent. It is certainly true of our feelings that whatever we are willing to experience *totally*, disappears. With luck, this may also turn out to be the case with your pain.

LISTEN TO SOOTHING MUSIC

Music is now known to help relieve pain. It has, for example, been successfully used at a Montreal hospital as a painkiller, and for facilitating childbirth at the Medical Center of the

University of Kansas. At the latter it was found that playing background music in the delivery room made labour easier, and that fewer painkilling drugs had to be used. In Poland a study of over 400 peopole suffering from migraine and various types of neurological illness revealed that those patients who listened regularly to music were able, after six months, to dispense with most of their drugs. A control group who did not listen to music still needed to take a full dose of painkillers to secure relief. The Appendix (page 143) lists some tapes of suitably relaxing music you might like to try.

While listening to music would be a good time to 'get down to Alpha' by practising the progressive body relaxation described in Chapter 3 on page 67.

RELIEVING MENTAL DISTRESS

The principle that what we are willing to allow ourselves to experience totally disappears can also be applied to mental distress. Continued bad feelings about something that happened in the past is a sure sign of what in Gestalt therapy is called 'unfinished business'. Our feelings, like our thoughts, will pass through us unless we are making them persist by clinging on to them. But there the similarity ends, for whereas going more deeply into thinking merely creates more thought for the inexhaustible mind, going more deeply into feelings discharges them for good.

Try this technique taken from Applied Kinesiology in order to complete the experience of some trauma that continues to haunt you. Place two fingers of each hand on the left and right 'bulges' of your forehead (frontal eminences) above the eyebrows. Maintain firm pressure without pressing too hard. Close your eyes and recall the situation that you found distressing at the time and still do. Re-run the mental video in as much detail as possible, at the same time allowing yourself to feel the emotions associated with the past experience as much as possible. Keep going over and over it until the energy has gone completely out of it. You will know when to stop when the images have faded so much it is hard to recall them any more. When you have worked through the trauma in this way, it should no longer return to trouble you.

THE CHAKRAS

To clear and balance blocked *chi* energy you could try meditating on the chakras (see below). The seven chakras are energy centres in the body associated with endocrine glands and nerve clusters. A diagram of the chakras is given on page 98. They are as follows:

CHAKRA	POSITION	CONTROLS
1st or 'root'	base of the spine	adrenals
2nd or 'sex'	above the genitals	gonads
3rd	solar plexus	pancreas
4th or 'heart'	cardiac plexus	thymus
5th	throat	thyroid
6th or 'third eye'	between the eyebrows	pituitary
7th or 'crown'	top of the head	pineal

Each of the seven chakras governs a certain type of energy that we use in our lives, and is associated with a certain colour, as follows;

CHAKRA	ENERGY TYPE	COLOUR
1st	survival; 'fight or flight'	red
2nd	social relating; sex	orange
3rd	power; independence; control	yellow
4th	love	green
5th	self-expression; authenticity	blue
6th	intuition, insight, awareness	indigo
7th	higher consciousness	violet

'Dis-ease' can manifest in any of the chakras, and

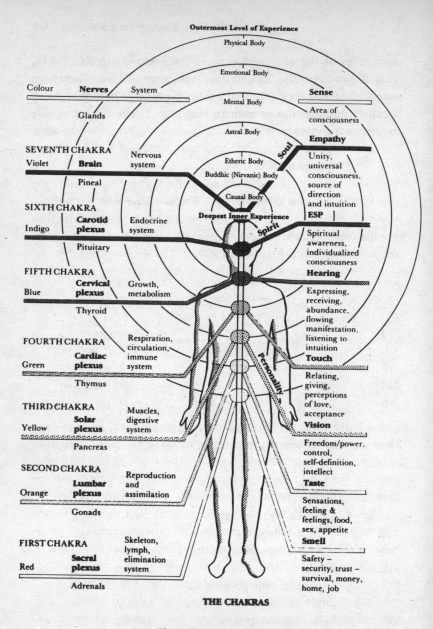

The Body–Mirror System.
Copyright © Martin Brofman, 1988.
After an illustration by Jørgen Høiland.

symptoms manifest in the area of the body controlled by it. This depends on the area of our lives in which we are experiencing stress, frustration or disappointment which is too much to handle on a conscious level, or of which we may be insufficiently aware. Meditating on the chakras in the way described below energizes them and clears blocked energy. It is both prophylactic and healing.

MEDITATION 19: HEALING THE CHAKRAS

TECHNIQUE

Working up progressively through the seven chakras, to cleanse and energize them and to unblock the energy coming through them.

This meditation can be done either sitting or lying. Let your attention rest in your first chakra at the base of the spine. Relax and breathe into this area. Allow yourself to feel any sensations that want to be experienced.

Start to visualize the colour red, in any way it comes: red curtains, a red scarf, or just a red haze. Continue to feel your first chakra as you create red in your mind's eye. Feel the lower part of your body starting to vibrate with this colour. Now visualize roots coming from the base of your spine and growing down your legs. Imagine these roots passing out through your feet and growing down into the earth. where they branch out into new roots. Allow yourself to feel deeply grounded, 'rooted'. After a while, imagine that you are drawing up into your body strength and energy through your roots. Feel this energy like molten lava flowing up slowly through your feet and legs and seeping into your spine. Enjoy the sensations and warmth and vitality this gives you.

When it feels right, move on to your second chakra. Let your attention rest on the pubis, just above the genitals. Once again, breathe into this area and tune into any sensations you may have there.

Now create in your mind the colour orange. It could be a bowl of oranges, an orange beach ball, the setting sun, or just an orange haze. In whatever form it comes, put the colour orange into the area of your second chakra.

Give yourself plenty of time. There is no hurry. Enjoy the colour orange for as long as you wish before moving up to the other chakras in turn. These, and the colours that energize them, are:

3rd	solar plexus	yellow
4th	heart	green
5th	throat	blue
6th	between the eybrows	indigo
7th	crown of the head	violet

Finish with Meditation 18: White Light (page 94), and make sure to ground yourself before resuming any activity.

TRANSFORMATION

Ikkyu, instead of writing 'attention, attention, attention', might just as well have written 'energy, energy, energy'. They are the same thing. Awareness and energy are aspects of the same coin, and meditation transforms them both, both quantitatively and qualitatively.

Becoming able to focus your attention where you want it to go, rather than, as usually happens, having it scattered all over the place by the many distractions surrounding us and clamouring for our attention, *conserves* energy. We leak it less, and feel less drained by being pulled here, there and everywhere. Giving ourselves space to be alone, sitting still and silent in a 'locked in' meditation posture, we allow our energy to build up again, and emerge from a session of resting in Alpha refreshed and recharged. We have seen earlier how such deep psychophysical relaxation increases our resistance to illness by strengthening our immunity, helps to heal us and make us feel better if we are sick or in pain.

As well as building up our energy when it is depleted, meditation also moves it up the chakras. Most people necessarily spend most of their time out in the world earning their living and relating, concerned with issues of survival, sex and staying in control of situations; so their energy mainly stays in the first three chakras. And most of the energy being beamed at us from newspapers, advertisements and films encourages us to think of the world in these terms. Our staple diet nightly on television, for example, consists largely of material dealing with politics, economics, crime and violence. When love is portrayed, it is usually in stereotyped ways and almost invariably linked with sexuality.

If we wish to move our energy up from these 'worldly' chakras in order to expand our consciousness, it would seem that we have to do it ourselves without much encouragement from our surroundings. Personal development is always an individual phenomenon. The larger the group, the more the 'herd mentality' and the lower the level of consciousness. Expanding our capacity for giving and receiving love (i.e. opening the heart chakra) is something we have to do for ourselves, as is finding out where our authenticity and creativity lie (fifth chakra) and risking expressing our individuality in the face, often, of social convention, expectations and judgements. Similarly, developing and learning to trust our intuition and insights (sixth chakra) is an ongoing process that comes only through constant dialogue with our inner self and 'Being a Light unto oneself'. And true spirituality (seventh chakra) is never a collective phenomenon. Our relationship to God, the Cosmos, Life, or however you perceive 'It', is always the most deeply personal and private relationship we have. To meditate is to act as midwife to your own birth process into higher consciousness. And though you may choose to meditate as a group in order to help raise the energy, what you do with it – and what it does to you – is a deeply personal experience. Enlightenment – the attainment of wholeness (holiness?), at-one-ment, self-realization or self-actualization, call it what you will – is always an individual phenomenon, yours and nobody else's.

Much has been written about the 'peak experiences' that sometimes occur when our psychic energy rises high enough above the more mundane levels of perceiving the world. These experiences can happen not only when we are doing formal meditation but also when we are in a 'meditative space', induced in us perhaps by being deeply moved by music or great art, or contemplating a beautiful view or sunset. Maslow has suggested that a peak experience tends to be triggered off by any experience of real excellence that absorbs our total attention and wonder. It could be anything that strikes a chord within us at a very deep level and with which our souls resonate as they are 'touched' by the perfection, the purity, beauty or sheer amazingness of whatever it is we are contemplating. It 'blows our minds' – an essential requisite for any experience of ecstasy.

A 'peak experience', as the term suggests, is a 'high' that may last for several minutes or several hours. Then it fades. Meditators who confuse a peak experience with enlightenment are discouraged by its disappearance and their return to a more prosaic level. 'What happened?' they say to themselves. 'Where did it go? It was so real . . .' Yes, it was real. But we must not cling on to experiences. We have to let go of them and allow room for the next one. They are graces for which we should be grateful, not greedy.

Beautiful as these peak experiences are, more valuable – because more permanent – are what Maslow calls 'plateau experiences'. These are shifts in our ways of perceiving and experiencing ourselves and the world from a deeper level of insight and feeling. Maslow himself describes how late in life, after his first heart attack, his awareness of the imminent possibility of death brought him a new appreciation and intensified awareness of the 'here and now'. This has been

the experience of many people who have survived cata-
strophic life-events, serious illness, perhaps, or loss. In retro-
spect they realize they have become more understanding and
capable of compassion, more grateful for the small things of
life and, perhaps above all, for the precious gift of life itself.
Happily, one can achieve a similar transformation of attitudes
and perception through meditation. It is even possible that
regular meditation helps one to 'burn up one's karma' so that
life does not have to jolt us into this deeper awareness by
putting us through such drastic learning experiences.

Regular meditation changes the *quality* of our energy. We
become softer, more sensitive. 'Opening the third eye' enables
us to see into our own hearts and into the hearts of others; to
see the truth behind the masks, façades and the games we
all play to protect the vulnerable child within. Opening our
heart chakra allows us to accept and love what we thus see,
without feeling we have to try to change others to make them
more perfect or how we think they should be (which usually
means: more like us). Don't bother; they are perfectly themselves already, and your only reward for not recognizing this
will be their resistance to your efforts to change them, if not
their outright hostility. In fact, unless we develop our heart
energies as well as our insight, the latter can be arid or even
destructive. It is not enough to see and share your insights
with others as to where they are 'at'. You have also to be
aware of whether or not they are strong enough to take what
you have to tell them, and whether or not they invited you to
share your insights in the first place.

Wisdom and compassion are like the two wings of a dove;
it needs both to be able to fly. One of the things that
sometimes discourages people from meditating is the arro-
gance of those who do, their subtly patronizing 'holier than
thou' attitude, their predilection for delivering little lectures
on higher consciousness at the drop of a hat, and playing
boring 'enlightenment games'. Fritz Perls, with his usual

bluntness, has classified much of our communication with each other as follows:

chicken shit: superficial, cocktail-party chatter;
bullshit: trying to impress the other person;
elephant shit: talking enlightened instead of being it.

Enjoy getting high during your meditation sessions. Learn from any peak experiences you may be blessed with, and the insights they bring. But don't get into an ego-trip about them. Keep them to yourself, treasure them as gifts from the universe helping you to higher consciousness. Don't (to use the jargon) 'blow the energy' – and you will get more where they came from.

6
STAYING CENTRED: MEDITATION IN THE MARKET-PLACE

Everything that happens to us, properly understood, leads us back to ourselves.

Jung

With practice, it becomes progressively easier to relax into the Alpha state when you are meditating in the privacy of your own home. Alas, only too often, as soon as we go out into the world again we lose our bliss and peace very quickly, ending up just as harassed, stressed and uptight as before. The 'Monday morning feeling' takes over and our lives become concerned with making ends meet or meeting expectations and deadlines. Rush, responsibility, pressure, tension . . . compounded by the sensory over-stimulation that surrounds and assails those of us who live and work in cities. How do we maintain the 'meditative space' in all this chaos? How do we stay centred, undisturbed, and on top of things?

In Chapter 2 we described the pathways to Alpha. They were:

witnessing
one-pointedness
listening
contemplation
present-centredness
awareness of breathing

body awareness
movement
centring.

Practising any one of these when you become aware of feeling fatigued, irritable or stressed will start to lower your level of Beta. If you are at work it may not be possible actually to go down to Alpha (except during breaks), for you will probably be using your left-side brain functions of concentrating, planning, discussing and so forth in the course of doing your job, which will keep you in the Beta brainwave range. But there is a difference between being in high Beta as a result of anxiety and other stress, and low Beta, the ordinary 'everyday' mind. Neither is particularly blissful (like Alpha), but at least low Beta is not likely to give you a nervous breakdown or a coronary, which staying habitually in high Beta might. And, of course, the more you slow down the more comfortable you will feel, as also will, probably, the people around you at work or with whom you have to deal, for tension is catching.

Let us take from these pathways to Alpha the 'knacks' that we can apply to stay meditative during our working day or whenever we find ourselves starting to wilt or tense up in 'the market-place'.

'Witnessing' really means 'detachment'. While it is good to be involved in what you are doing rather than distracted and bored, you can become *too* involved at an ego-level. The more attached you are to results, the more perfectionist, the more out to impress the boss, the more tense you will become. Unless you remain in touch with yourself as the 'doer' *while* you are doing what you do, you will tend to be easily 'thrown' when things go wrong or do not turn out the way you wanted them to. You will have given your power away to something outside yourself which may bring you down and affect your mood, instead of 'staying in charge'. However hectic the pace, however intense the concentration demanded by your job, try to keep a sense of who you are, *who* is doing this job.

KNACKS FOR STAYING CENTRED

1. *Stay in touch with your feelings* as well as with the outer reality. Tune in every so often to how you are feeling, e.g. bored, impatient, hungry. Note your feeling without judgement or trying to change it.

2. Remind yourself from time to time of the action in which you are engaged by *naming* it to yourself, e.g. 'writing, writing'.

3. *Be aware of when you are starting to leak energy* by too much effort or unnecessary talking, and 'pull your energy back in'. A lot of energy is expended through the eyes, so try not to be distracted by things (or people) clamouring for your attention (unless, of course, it's your boss!).

4. *Give yourself 'breathing space'.* Take a break from concentrating every so often and become aware of how you may be restricting your breathing through tension. Take a few deep breaths. Look around the room at people, furniture, objects, to ground yourself and bring you back to the present.

5. *Become aware again of your body and body sensations.* Stretch, go for a little walk to the washroom. Feel your feet on the floor. Rub your hands together . . .

6. *'Come to your senses'* in any way you can. Listen to sounds (without identifying them). Contemplate and enjoy the fragrance of any flowers in the room, or appreciate in detail a picture on the wall. Feel an object on your desk (paperweights are particularly pleasant to play with). If in the washroom, soak your hands and wrists in water as hot as you can bear (this is very calming).

7. *Above all, be here now!*

HOW TO KEEP YOUR COOL WHEN OTHERS ARE LOSING THEIRS

One of the times when we are liable to wish that we *weren't* here now is when we are engaged in some sort of confrontation with another person. None of us likes to be criticized or told off. Most of us find our own anger hard to handle and are threatened by other people's. All of us want to feel liked and approved of. What do you do when the adrenalin is beginning to rise and, worst of all, when the person who is giving you a bad time is somebody that you have to take it easy with: your boss or a client, for example; your querulous invalid mother who may be living with you; or the teenage rebel in your classroom who can be such a provocative pain in the neck?

What you can do is to counteract the contraction that occurs whenever you feel threatened, halt the release of adrenalin that goes with the 'fight or flight' response and try to remain centred. Here's how.

1. *Breathe.* We tend to stop breathing if we are shocked in any way.

2. *Feel your feet on the floor.* 'Stand your ground.'

3. *Maintain an open body posture.* Uncross your arms and legs, unclench your fists. We can often change the way we feel by changing our body posture (e.g. in yoga). The more you contract your body muscles the more tense and threatened you will feel.

4. *Contemplate the other person.* What does an angry person look like? Note the frown or scowl, the tightness in the jaw, the jerky movements and perhaps gesticulations. 'Just watching' will shift your awareness from involvement in trying to defend or excuse yourself to the position of witness – and thus puts space between you.

5. *Listen.* Try to tune into the place the other person is coming from. Behind the angry words, what are they really feeling? What 'button' has been pushed? If the other feels

that he or she is really being *heard*, what usually happens is that they will calm down.

6. *Respond* to the place the other is coming from, rather than reacting to their words, or from your own panic or need to please.

7. *Stay in touch* with what is going on with you during this transaction. Don't accept put-downs under any circumstances. If you feel invalidated or misjudged, say so. You may have been at fault in some way, but you are always deserving of respect.

RELATIONSHIP QUARRELS

More upsetting than anything that goes on 'in the market-place' are the confrontations that take place in the privacy of our own homes. The stoical detachment we may be able to maintain during office or similar crises tends to crumble when we find ourselves on the receiving end of recrimination or blaming (or, even worse, sulking), or when we ourselves are angered by something our partner said or did.

Most often, quarrels between people living together arise from confusion about *space*. There is a natural rhythm in all of us: at times we want to be together and at other times we need to be alone, 'in our own space'. In relationships, too, a dynamic is usually present of 'togetherness' versus 'individuality'. Part of us wants to merge with the other person, another part fears becoming too dependent and losing a sense of self. Irritation with one's partner is very often about experiencing the other as either withholding or intrusive, either because they are not being sensitive to our need for intimacy, or to our need for privacy.

How does meditation help us to sweeten our relationships and to make them more harmonious?

1. It makes us more sensitive to *energy*. We become more 'in tune' with the vibrations our partner is putting out, whether of the 'I want to get closer' or the 'I want some

space' variety. Moving with the changing energy between you makes for harmony — and fun; trying to impose your own needs without regard for the other, doesn't.

2. Sitting quietly in meditation teaches us to appreciate the beauty of *silence* and to feel comfortable with it. Many spouses and lovers are driven to distraction by the constant chattering of their partners. This is often an attempt to avoid silence (experienced as vaguely threatening) or real communication (which often arises out of silence which has allowed us to feel 'where we are at', rather than half-listening to superficial chatter). 'Talking about' (and especially talking about the past or the future, or people who are not present) takes us away from the here and now as nothing else does. It is only in this present moment that we really meet, and often words get in the way.

3. Meditation makes us more *self-sufficient*. As we learn how to nourish ourselves at a very deep level we become less 'needy', less dependent on others to 'make us feel good'. Many people are constantly trying to fill the inner emptiness, like a hole inside them that they are dimly aware of, by compulsive eating. Some devour food; others 'devour' people. We say they 'suck' energy, are 'leeches'. These are the clingers, the clamourers for attention, the wanters. But no one person can ever fill all your needs, even supposing they wanted to, and they are not here to meet your expectations either. Unless we develop our inner resources and learn to nourish ourselves (as in meditation), not only will we have a hard time feeling we are in an equal relationship and often feel rejected or over-dependent, but we may well drive our partner away through our constant demands and neediness. Perhaps we have to learn to be alone before we can truly be in a relationship without disempowering ourselves and losing our sense of who we are. Meditation is about enjoying your aloneness, and is an antidote to *loneliness*.

LISTENING TO OUR SELVES

Meditating regularly puts us more in touch with our selves, the various different parts of us that make us who we are, and thus has much in common with psychotherapy. Sitting watching our thoughts, listening to the inner dialogue that goes on ceaselessly, we come to recognize certain 'voices' within us that surface over and over again. They are really patterns of energy, specific and more or less fixed, in our unconscious, akin to the belief systems that are like programs in our mind-computer. They are *habits of being*, habitual ways of responding and expressing ourselves, and they take over our consciousness whenever they are activated.

Jung called these unconscious patterns 'complexes'. Bringing them into the light of ego-consciousness forms a large part of most forms of psychotherapy, for as long as we remain unconscious of them we have little control over them. They manipulate our thinking and our feeling, impel us to act out or to act in, and to react in ways that sometimes we blush to remember. In short, they 'pull our strings', making us react always in the same way in similar types of situations.

Modern psychotherapists have called these different parts of us 'subpersonalities' because they really do behave as if they were real and separate people inside us. And, verily, we are a crowd. Here are some subpersonalities that we all have.

The Parent. The Parent within us has two aspects, to nurture and to protect. In its zeal to protect us – and others – it can be very controlling, just like a real parent. The Parent is the part that likes to 'lay down the law' and tries to enforce obedience to its notion of right and wrong. It is also the part that is capable of caring, nourishing ourselves and others, being responsible and a 'good citizen'.

The Inner Critic. Like the Parent, the Inner Critic is an introjection of the expectations of the authority figures of our childhood – the parents, teachers, priests, etc., who had very firm ideas on how we should behave and the standards we should try to attain. It is therefore akin to our 'conscience'. This is the part of us that is continually reminding us of our inadequacies, and, if sufficiently sadistic, can wreck our confidence and self-esteem. The voice of the Critic is instantly recognizable, for it likes to deliver little lectures to us on how we 'should' be. Its positive aspect is that it 'keeps us up to scratch' and stops us behaving so badly that we could end either with no friends or in jail.

The Pleaser. The Pleaser is the part of us that wants always to be liked, and will do almost anything to avoid unpleasantness, confrontation, or criticism. If you have a highly-developed Pleaser you will sell yourself short to please the other, say 'Yes' when you really mean 'No', and never ask for what you want in case the other doesn't approve. On the other hand, if you have a well-developed Pleaser, you will never be short of friends, for he (or she) makes you easy to be with.

The Driver. If you have taken up meditation because you are a workaholic and have been told you have to ease up, this is the subpersonality you need to get to know better. And you will, because when you sit in meditation the Driver's voice will come through loud and clear, telling you what a waste of time this is, and reminding you of all the things that need to be done. The Driver is the most unmeditative of all subpersonalities. It is the 'doer' in all of us: it wants results, is always in a rush, and always finding more things that need doing. It is probably responsible for more coronaries than any other single factor, for it creates stress. On the other hand, it does get things done.

The Inner Child. However old we get, we never lose the Child within us. It is our capacity for openness, playfulness, spontaneity and wonder, and also our capacity to *feel*, which makes it very vulnerable. Many people have stifled the Child within them as a defence against this vulnerability, to avoid being disappointed or hurt. The more hard, unfeeling, cynical or sophisticated the façade they put up to protect the Child within, the more deeply wounded it must have been – and the more needing of nurturing. It is no accident that so much of the work in psychotherapy is to do with childhood experience, and the relaxing of rigidity and recovery of feeling and spontaneity that attends successful therapy is akin to rescuing the Inner Child from its isolation and letting it out to play.

These are only some of the subpersonalities we all have. There are very many more, and readers interested in finding out more about them can do so from my *Who's Pulling your Strings?* (Thorsons, 1989).

Being able to recognize at any one time which of our personalities is taking over our consciousness and influencing our emotions and actions is useful if we wish to 'stay in charge' and not be carried away by our feelings and stampeded into doing or saying things we may later regret. We need, for example, to be aware when our Workaholic is taking over and making us over-extend ourselves; when our Pleaser is making us commit ourselves to things we would rather not do, simply because we shrink from saying what we really want. We need to be able to recognize the Inner Critic's harsh judgements of us and tell it to shut up, rather than allowing it to bring us down and feel bad about ourselves. Above all, we need to be in touch with the needs of our Inner Child, to nurture it and respect our own sensitivity and vulnerability rather than labelling it as 'weakness'.

'Staying cool' in an argument or quarrel is very much easier if one becomes aware of how the subpersonalities are polarized. The most recent and sophisticated method of working with these subpersonalities, Voice Dialogue, was hit upon by its founders, American psychoanalyst Dr Hal Stone and his wife Dr Sidra Winkelman, as a result of a domestic quarrel. At a certain point in their quarrel, she became aware that her husband seemed to have regressed to being a child again: plaintive, sulky, vulnerable. She abandoned what we all usually do in quarrels – defending herself and counter-attacking – and instead assumed the role of Good Mother, dropping the one of Rebellious Daughter that she had been playing in response to her projections on her husband of Controlling Father. The change in the energy between them was immediate and startling. Hal's Child, sensitive to the change in Sidra, now felt able to share the unfulfilled needs that were really behind his blaming and complaining. Sidra, no longer feeling under attack, could now be centred enough to listen to the hurt and need her husband was really expressing and respond to that rather than to his angry words. (*Embracing Our Selves* by Hal Stone and Sidra Winkelman (Devorss and Co., 1985).)

Don't assume that you have to get angry just because the other person is angry with you. Be aware of your tendency to project on to the other the Bad Parent and then to oppose it as Rebellious Son or Daughter; or when your own Controlling Parent is laying down the law and driving your partner deeper into their Child. The sooner you can become aware of the hurt behind the anger, the insecurity behind the jealousy, the need behind the demand, the sooner you will be addressing real issues in your relationship, rather than merely playing ping-pong and putting your energy into scoring points.

7
THINKING CREATIVELY

Planners make canals, archers shoot arrows,
craftsmen fashion woodwork, the wise man moulds
himself.

Dhammapada

One of the bonuses of regular meditation is detachment from identification with the thought process. Witnessing our thoughts coming and going, we learn new ways of relating to them. No longer do we feel impelled to follow every train of thought that happens to be passing through our heads. We can take them or leave them. And, if we decide to leave them, we are spared the feelings that are spawned by them. For feelings follow thoughts, and if we nip a depressing thought in the bud we interrupt the normal process by which, unchecked, it burgeons into feelings that we then may feel impelled to act out. Through regular meditation, we become sufficiently aware of our thinking process to become its masters and not its slaves. We can choose which thoughts to give attention to, and which to ignore and let subside again into the nothingness from which they came.

Attention is *energy*. What we give attention to becomes more manifest in our world. Everything starts as thought. Consider, for example, how the house you are living in came to be there. It had its origins in a project in somebody's mind – a builder or a property developer. Considering a house on this site to be a 'good idea' (i.e. to be worth thinking more about) he engages an architect with whom he discusses (i.e.

exchanges ideas about, feeds more attention to) the form the house should take (i.e. how it should manifest on the physical plane). As soon as the architect starts to draw up his plans, already the energy that between them they are feeding into the project becomes denser and starts to manifest on the material plane. What was merely an idea is beginning to 'take shape'. As the project gathers momentum, the builder's men move on to the site and pour their energy into making a house materialize there: bricklayers, carpenters, glaziers, plumbers, electricians – all add their energy. Eventually, where there had been empty space, the house now stands, the embodiment of the original idea. Unless, that is, other ideas with sufficient power to interrupt or abort the process of creation supervene: for example, a petition by local residents against the project or refusal of planning permission by the Town Hall.

Thought is creative. What we have said about the process by which your house came to exist is true of everything in the manifested world: cities, artefacts, literature, art, crime – they all started as ideas in somebody's head and were thought worth making a reality by 'working on them'. 'Working on' means 'giving energy to'.

We create our reality by what we choose to give our attention to. Attention energizes, makes more real. We start to talk about it (the first stage of manifestation) and to act out our feelings about it (the second stage). It is an awesome thought that we are creating our future by what we are thinking, feeling and saying now. These are seeds that we are planting that will surely, sooner or later, bear fruit in the objective world. Whether we end up choked by a jungle of weeds or enjoying a beautiful garden is up to us.

Life is impartial. It is very respectful of our freedom to choose our creations, almost as if it were more interested in the creative process itself rather than actually what we create. One thinks inevitably of Hitler. For example, it supports whatever we are prepared to believe about ourselves. We get more of 'where we are at', and more 'juice' for our projects.

Psychologists have found that our perception of the world, 'the way things are', is highly selective. We see whatever happens through the filter of our belief systems, what we expect to see. In other words, our minds project on to the world pictures that are inside us about how it is, and we then feel and act according to these pictures. The world is thus like a mirror: we are always seeing ourselves, our attitudes, desires, expectations, reflected in it. In this sense, our world is always our own creation and there are as many worlds as there are people. *Quot homines, tot sententiae.*

When we are dissatisfied with our world (or, as they say in America, 'our lives are not working') normally what we do is try to change the outer reality in some way. We may move house, get a new job, separate or divorce and so on. But, more often than not, we find ourselves after the novelty has worn off re-creating the same situations, the same boredom and frustration, making the same mistakes. And inevitably so, for we take ourselves with us when we move. Unless we work to change the patterns of thinking that are like blueprints for experiencing and for action inside us, nothing changes. We just go on repeating. And this is true in the case of our health as well. It is increasingly being seen, for example, that habitual negative mental patterns like resentment or guilt can help to create illness in our bodies, cancer for example. Well-documented and sometimes dramatic cases of remission or cure have occurred when the patient has decided to let go of such negative patterns, to forgive and forget. Without this change in the mental patterns that helped to manifest the physical pattern of illness in the body, surgery or chemotherapy may remove one cancer only for the patient to re-create it, perhaps in another part of the body. This is a model of what happens in other areas of our lives as well, in our relationships, for example. We go on getting involved with the same sort of person, playing the same power games, experiencing the same jealousy and possessiveness, walking out of the relationship at the same point. Merely changing our partner doesn't help. *Plus ça change, plus c'est la même chose.*

In meditation, rather than struggling to change our *outer* reality, we try to become aware of how we create it and keep it in existence: our habitual ways of thinking and seeing, what we tell ourselves about 'the way it is' – and we are – that make us experience the world and ourselves in the way we do. Change the inner and the outer follows, for the latter is merely mirroring what is inside us. When we change our belief systems our experience of the world changes with them. In this way meditation is rather like a self-help psychotherapy based on insight into our self-limiting and self-destructive patterns. It has the added advantage of enabling us to detach ourselves sufficiently from acting out these patterns to develop the capacity to witness our own behaviour rather than being trapped in it.

Watching our minds in meditation reminds us that we always have a choice as to what we think about. If we are centred in ourselves, nobody can force us to think anything, let alone *feel* anything. One of the biggest manipulations of all is to be told, or to tell someone else: 'You made me feel bad' (guilty, angry, etc.). Nobody has that power. But it is also true that from a very early age we are conditioned to accept the thought-forms of others, e.g. our parents, teachers and peers, in order ourselves to be accepted by them. We chose to introject their value judgements and belief systems, simply because not to do so would be to court disapproval, or punishment, perhaps even jeopardize our survival.

Some of our conditioning is, of course, necessary to allow us to survive and move in the world. It is useful to know, for example, that you have to look both ways before crossing the road, or that good manners are more likely than bad to make us socially acceptable. Learning to read and write opens up many possibilities for us, while being trained for a job enables us to achieve independence and, we hope, enjoy our own creativity. But along with this necessary and useful conditioning, we take in less valuable ways of behaving and seeing that perhaps do not fit us as well as they did the people who passed them on to us. Also, as a result of things that happen to us in the process of growing up, we ourselves come to certain conclusions about how we should behave in future. We may have told ourselves things like, 'I'm never going to do that again', or 'People are not to be trusted' (only interested in you for what they can get out of you, around only as long as they need you, etc.).

Our minds are rather like computers, and our conditioning, either from others or from the conclusions we ourselves draw from our life experiences, is stored in them as programs. We have many, many programs, and the vast majority of them are unconscious ones. We simply forget our original choice to see things in this particular way. We store away conclusions about life which then become more or less rigid belief systems that control the way we think, the sorts of things we think about, how we feel about ourselves and others. The more we are identified with these beliefs, the more rigid they become – and the more threatened we feel if they are challenged in any way. When our ideas are attacked it feels as if we ourselves are being attacked. The more threatened we feel, the more the anger (or the loss of self-esteem or the depression, which is anger turned inwards). This is what quarrelling is about; it is as true on the global as on the individual scale. Countries will go to war to defend a sense of identity that is inextricably associated with a particular religion, political bias or economic system. Within the state, this takes the form of persecution of minorities, censorship and other kinds of repression. The world will be a more peaceful and harmonious place once we get the double message: first, that our belief systems should support us, not the other way round; and, second, that they are moveable feasts.

Belief systems that are not subject to revision, modification – or cannot simply be let go of – become like straitjackets. They limit our freedom of action and effectively bar the way to freshness of experience and personal growth. It has been said that it is not what ideas we have that make us mad, but the degree of obsessiveness with which we cling to them. To remain mentally healthy we have to learn how to tolerate the paradoxes and contradictions of life, rather than trying to impose our own one-sided views on it and struggling to maintain them. And a struggle it will surely be, for the opposite is always there. And the more we try to annihilate it and deny its existence, the more energy it gathers and the more we will find ourselves confronted by it in our daily lives. For peaceful co-existence, it is essential to be able to tolerate *difference*.

What we resist, persists. For every component of our ego-consciousness, there is the corresponding opposite energy in our unconscious to balance it. Much of psychotherapy, especially the assimilation of the Shadow in Jungian analytical psychology, is about bringing material that has been repressed because it did not 'fit' with conscious attitudes into the light of ego-awareness and encouraging the patient to 'hold the opposites'. Unless this is done, the individuation (self-actualizing) process cannot happen. The repressed alternative ways of being and thinking remain as complexes out of conscious control, to sabotage our best intentions and make us neurotic. We are constantly disturbed by them, for any energies that we disown in ourselves become projected outwards into the world and attract the same type of energy to us. Thus we will constantly be running up against people 'out there' who embody the very things we disapprove of yet are unconscious of in ourselves. We will be haunted by any energy that we are unwilling to honour in ourselves, and not only by day. Dreams are the attempts of the psyche to achieve balance by integrating the bits of ourselves that we have disowned: they are messages from the unconscious to our ego-consciousness that our conscious attitudes are too rigid, too exclusive. The less we heed them, the more nightmarish they can become.

There is a saying in zen: 'Let the mind have no abiding-place.' One of the tricks of the mind is to persuade us that we have found the truth, that we have 'got it', once and for all. But in fact all we have 'got', however exciting or beautiful the insight, is relative. It may be true now, but perhaps tomorrow it will be true no longer. For truth is not something fixed, but an ongoing and ever-changing experience, like Life itself. The real truth lies in experiencing moment to moment what is real for us *now*. Not only is truth not an idea that can be expressed in words; words in fact get in the way of our experience of it. As Lao-Tzu puts it in the *Tao Te Ching*: 'The Tao that can be told is not the eternal Tao' (ch. 1); and again, 'He who knows, does not speak. He who speaks, does not know' (ch. 56).

Meditation rescues us from the tyranny of concepts *about* the world and ourselves and trains us in the art of experiencing the latter directly, wordlessly. Resisting the mind's obsession with labelling everything and wanting to put it into a neat little category – and thereby thinking it 'knows' it – means tolerating 'not knowing'. Paradoxically, we have to drop knowledge to experience truth.

It may seem to the reader from the foregoing that we are invalidating the marvellous capacity we human beings have evolved for thought. But in fact what we have been stressing is the sheer *power* of thought and the necessity for harnessing this power creatively so that it works for us instead of against us. Thought is energy. Like other forms of energy, it can enhance the quality of our lives or wreck them. Electricity, for example, can (literally) lighten our lives, be used to cook a delicious meal, or inflict horrible burns. Water can quench our thirst, or drown us. Energy is neutral, and it is our responsibility to use it wisely. Similarly with thought: we can direct it creatively or be made tense, unhappy or even driven mad by it when it is unchecked. Meditation is the only way to achieve the detachment from the thought process itself and the one-pointedness which are necessary prerequisites for bringing the wayward mind to heel so that it can serve us rather than control us. Once we have meditated sufficiently to realize that we are the thinker and not the thinking process, we are then in a position from which to choose what to think, and how to think about it. Let us look now at some of the ways in which we can think creatively, and create more quality in our lives.

MEDITATING ON THE OPPOSITE

This is simply a technique to counteract a negative frame of mind by deliberately dwelling on its opposite, positive counterpart. For example, if we are angry with somebody, instead of fuelling the anger by re-running the quarrel or hurt in our heads we can choose to forgive them and direct loving thoughts towards them (see the *Metta* meditation on pages 89–91). By doing this we avoid stressing ourselves by either acting out or repression. We neither hurt the other person, nor risk poisoning our bodies (and especially our immune systems) by holding on to resentments. If you think this may be hard, remember that being willing to forgive is enough to halt the descent into more anger and to stop the adrenalin flowing. And to forgive is not the same as condoning or colluding with the way the other may have treated you. What you are choosing to do is to love yourself enough not to let yourself continue to be disturbed by whatever happened, and to restore your peace of mind. At your next meeting you may well want to confront the person with his or her behaviour and will be able to do this more calmly and objectively. Rather than attacking or blaming, which usually provokes counter-attack and defensiveness, you may well be more inclined this time round to share with the other person how you felt hurt by what they said or did, which is less threatening for them, and may well elicit an apology.

CHANGING OLD PATTERNS

As we said before, nobody can *make* us feel anything. If we get angry, it is *our* anger, and we alone are responsible for dealing with it. Most of us carry around anger from the past, from unfinished situations, for example with our parents. This anger can be triggered off (or, in the jargon of humanistic psychology, our 'button pushed') by situations that remind us of the original anger-producing incidents way back. For example, we may be projecting on our spouse the withholding mother of our childhood, or our authoritarian father. When they say 'No' to us, we may react as if we were still children rebelling against being told what to do and what not to do.

Unless we become aware of this rebellious side to us and that we are carrying around with us a 'button' just waiting to be pushed, people will be pushing it all the time, without either knowing they are doing so, or even intending to. And each time we will react in a robot-like fashion, getting angry time and time again whenever the button is pushed.

This is not to say that we should not acknowledge our anger. Quite the contrary: all of our feelings, whatever they are, should always be honoured. But this is not the same as saying that we should allow them to control us like puppets on a string, reacting automatically in this or that way whenever this or that string is pulled. The way to unhook yourself from the string is through insight. First of all become aware that the pattern exists. Meditate on it, get to know the mechanism of stimulus and reaction intimately and exactly how it feels. See what images come to mind from the past, what associations. Observe yourself in action, and when you start to get angry, note the fact. Deliberately check yourself from following the same old pattern of reacting. Choose this time to respond in a different way for a change. For the first few times you may fail in your intention of not rising to the same bait and getting 'hooked'. Don't blame yourself: at least now you are aware you are doing so and taking responsibility for your own anger rather than blaming others for 'making you angry' and thus casting yourself in a victim role.

It sounds hard, but the more you experience the freedom and relief from dropping old patterns of negativity the easier it gets. For the process is merely that of letting go of old, stale ideas – but ideas that still have the power to generate disturbing feelings in you. Once you get the hang of it, you will be actively on the watch in your daily life for evidence of patterns that need dropping. Signs to watch for include the rigidity of your judgements, feeling hurt by anything somebody else says or does, getting disturbed when your expectations are not met, or the compulsive brooding on a situation that is a sure sign of 'unfinished business'. And remember to be grateful to anybody who 'pushed your buttons'. If they hadn't, you might not have known they were there. In this sense, everybody is our teacher. And once the button is processed and removed through insight, the button-pushers also disappear, because you will no longer be attracting them into your energy field.

VISUALIZATION

Our experience can be changed by changing our mental pictures. Our bodies do not distinguish between imagined reality and 'real', in the sense of objective reality. It will obligingly produce the set of feelings and physiological responses to match the picture being exhibited on our mental screens. If these pictures are negative, *angst*-laden or scary, our 'fight or flight' response will be activated in the same way as if we were actually being confronted by these situations in real life. We (and that includes our bodies) respond to what we *believe* to be true. Also, as we have suggested, attention is energy: dwelling on something constantly in our minds tends to make it more manifest in our lives by attracting energy of a similar type to us from outside. To visualize is to make conscious use of this mechanism in order to end up feeling the way we would like to feel – i.e. good – rather than being stuck with the all-too-often negative or uncomfortable moods imposed on us by our minds. Here are a few you might like to try.

BEFORE STARTING A NEW PROJECT

Imagine yourself engaged in the project, doing marvellously, in as much detail as possible. Imagine that the project has been successfully completed to your total satisfaction. Get the feeling in your body of joy and a sense of fulfilment. Create in your mind's eye celebrating your success, and receiving the congratulations of those close to you. Enjoy this fantasy for as long as you wish. This visualization gears you for success, gives you confidence and optimism, and will therefore affect positively the way you present yourself to others who can help further your project, e.g. bank managers, potential employers or backers.

DISPELLING FEAR

Imagine 'fear' as a black cloud that is hovering above your head. It is attached to you by a string. Visualize yourself cutting this string and thus releasing the cloud. Watch it as it rises higher and higher and eventually disappears into the sky. Feel the relief in your body, the lightening-up as tension disappears with the balloon.

ANXIETY ABOUT MONEY

Worrying about lack of money will only make your situation

worse. The messages you are thus broadcasting to the universe are, 'I am a beggar and I do not trust in the Abundance of the Universe and that I shall always have enough.' And that experience is exactly what you will get more of. Remember that life tends to provide us with the evidence to justify our own belief systems. If you choose to identify with being a beggar you will be geared to see 'lack' wherever you look, filtering out from your perception all the ways in which in fact you are provided for, and certainly have more than the majority of people on this planet.

Change the messages you are broadcasting. Instead of worrying about not having enough, look at what you *do* have. Substitute prosperity-consciousness in place of your poverty-consciousness. Visualize yourself as already having everything you want. How would that feel? How would you be living differently to the way you are now? Meditate on the abundance of the universe that surrounds us if only we look: 'Consider the lilies of the field, how they grow; they toil not, neither do they spin.' Meditate on 'trust'. Most important of all, act as if you are already prosperous and thank the universe for what it has bestowed on you. Acting 'as if' is a powerful device for attracting to you the experiences you desire. Money attracts money. A well-heeled friend of mine told me once that the more wealthy you are, the more other people are ready to give you things: free services, personal attention, credit. I remember as he spoke thinking of the beggars in India when I lived there: their desperation, the outstretched hands, and the often-expressed irritation or indifference of passers-by. Think of yourself as a beggar and the world will treat you like one.

It could also be a good idea to meditate on your patterns about money. Very few of us are clear in this important area of our lives. Many people, for example, get embarrassed at being asked to name a price for something they are selling, and undersell themselves. Others find it hard to ask for money that has been borrowed by another and held on to for too long. If, therefore, you are experiencing the energy we call money as not exactly flowing in your direction, it might be a good idea to meditate on how perhaps you may be blocking the flow by your belief-systems about it. When you do look into your conditioning about money and how you relate to it these are some of the 'tapes' you might find you have stored away in your mind-computer:

Money is hard to come by.
Other people get rich, not me.
You really have to work hard to get money.
To want money is 'uncool' and very bourgeois.
Unless I have a lot of money life is not worth living.
If I get more, others will have less.

Any such tape is very easily changed by substituting another which says the exact opposite – and thus cancels it out. One way to do this is with Affirmations.

AFFIRMATIONS

Affirmations are statements that we deliberately feed into our mind-computers to reprogram ourselves for more quality of life. If we repeat them often enough, they sink like seeds deep into our subconscious, where they germinate and eventually start to sprout and bear fruit in our lives as positive experiences. We make use of the mechanism that, alas, works so well in the case of political propaganda: repeat a slogan often enough and people start to act as if it were true.

Use affirmations whenever in your insight meditations you come across a tape that is limiting you in any way, if not actively sabotaging you and your projects. For example: with regard to the self-limiting program about money listed above, affirmations to antidote them could run as follows:

Money is easy to come by.
I deserve to be wealthy.

Money naturally follows the project. I don't have to kill myself
    for it.
It's OK to want money and the security, comfort and the goodies
    it can bring.
Money is my servant: it is here to serve me.
There is enough to go round.

Affirmations should be repeated at intervals during the
day, at least twice on each occasion, when we are relaxed
enough to allow them to sink in. The best time for making
them is immediately on waking in the morning or last thing
at night before falling asleep. It could also reinforce their
power to shorten them to one or two words and to use this
as a mantra more often. Examples of this could be repeating
'Abundance, Abundance', or 'Prosperity, Prosperity' (a little
more elegant perhaps than 'Money, Money'!).

IMPROVED SELF-IMAGE AND CONFIDENCE

Affirmations are particularly effective in counteracting one of
the most damaging things our minds can inflict on us,
namely, telling us that we are inadequate in some way. The
Perfectionist and the Critic inside us can be quite sadistic,
and one wonders how many people have been made seriously
depressed or even driven to suicide by these inner voices
repeatedly telling them that they are no good.

So whenever you catch yourself putting yourself down,
blaming or invalidating yourself in any way whatsoever,
cancel these negative and potentially toxic tapes by telling
yourself the contrary.

I love and approve of myself totally, every moment.
It's OK to feel the way I do.
I do not have to be perfect.
I forgive myself totally for . . .
I accept myself completely, just as I am, right now.

Once again, combine positive statements with an awareness of the patterns of negativity about yourself that you have taken on board somewhere along the way. Listen to the voice of your Inner Critic carefully. Whose voice does it remind you of from your past? What images come to mind from your childhood? Whose expectations are you trying to meet by putting pressure on yourself to be different from how you are?

Affirmations and visualizations are examples of what is called 'Meditation with seed' (i.e. content), as opposed to 'Meditation without seed' which is meditation of the purely witnessing type, such as *vipassana* and *zazen*. Prayer is also an example of 'meditation with seed'. And, in fact, affirmations and visualizations are akin to prayer in that you are sending messages out to the universe asking for help, and trusting that you will be heard.

Do not discuss what you are doing with anybody else. The process of thinking creatively is, as we have said, akin to planting seeds – and seeds need to be left undisturbed to germinate in the fertile darkness of the earth. Do not allow yourself to get into ego-trips when the fruits start to manifest in your life, as they surely will. These are graces bestowed on you by a benevolent universe and the appropriate response is gratitude.

8
SELF-REMEMBERING

*Everyone is the Self, and indeed is infinite. Yet each
person mistakes his body for his Self.*

Ramana Maharshi

We usually take up meditation in order to relax
more and to lessen the stress in our lives; this it certainly
does by rescuing us from the tyranny of the restless mind,
withdrawing our attention from being fragmented and scattered by the Ten Thousand Things and centring it instead in
our own Self. It is a 180 degree turn: from looking outside
our selves, to looking inside at our own process; from being
pulled out into involvement in the outer, to resting in the
peace and stillness of the 'centre of the cyclone'. Meditation
is to exchange the role of the doer for that of the witness.

As we practise meditation more and more, we become
calmer, less easily disturbed by what is going on around us.
We feel more empowered to create what we want out of life
(instead of being stuck with what we get) by having regained
control over our attention. We can decide to have more of
this in our lives and less of that, by feeding attention and
energy, or withdrawing it (and, especially, by not leaking it).
We come to realize that life is always mirroring us, and that
if our lives are not working it is up to us to put our house in
order, to change the inner, rather than blaming others or
outside influences. If we are willing to accept responsibility
for the choices we make (or made in the past) we move from
the position of victim to taking charge of our lives. In the
process we become more in touch with our bodily, emotional

and spiritual needs, what we want – and what we don't want.

As we become more sensitive to our own process it becomes harder for us to act against what we really feel. Our relationships deepen (either that, or we grow out of them) as we become less interested in the games and role-playing, the striving to impress that make up much of our social inter-action. We become more authentic, simply because it is more satisfying to be the person we are rather than the person whom others would like us to be. And as we develop a taste for the freedom that follows our release from the straitjacket of conditioning and false identifications, we become more will-ing to co-operate with the process of understanding that we embarked upon, whether deliberately or not, when we decided to become meditators. We become *interested* in under-standing our own negativity and its origins, and in working to transform it, rather than being appalled by it and shoving it under the carpet with denial, repression and projecting it on to others. Everything becomes grist to the mill of our awareness, and every situation a learning experience, remind-ing us of the areas in which there is still 'unfinished business'.

Meditation changes us, so be prepared! It is not so much that we become different, but that we become who we always were. The process has been likened to remembering what has been forgotten, buried under conditioning and false identifications that we gradually slough off like an old skin the more we investigate who we really are. The experi-ence of finding the self again is always deeply satisfying – and somehow familiar. It has been likened to feeling as free, fresh and innocent as a child again, yet with the added awareness from all the living we have done since we were children. The more we meditate the more often these experi-ences come, although, alas, they tend to fade as we get caught up again in our old habits. It was to avoid the latter that, in the East, seekers after enlightenment (*sannyasins*) would, in middle age when they had satisfied social and marital obligations, withdraw from the world to devote all their energy to meditation. From a different point of view, this is also what contemplatives in the religious orders in the West have done.

The deeper one goes into meditation, the more blurred the boundaries become between it, religion and psychotherapy. For they all have in common the search for inner truth, the return to authentic being and the healing of our inner psychic wounds. We tend to regard religions as belief-systems. Yet their founders have in fact been masters showing us the 'way back' to *experiencing* who we really are and had a zen-like scorn for purely intellectual knowledge. Witness Jesus' condemnation of the Pharisees, and his words: 'Except ye be converted [i.e. transform your consciousness] and become as little children, ye shall not enter into the kingdom of heaven.' We are not to be childish, but *children*: for as well as being 'innocent as doves' we have also to be 'wise as serpents' (i.e. aware). Buddha's last words, as he lay dying, to his brother Anand were: 'Be a Light unto Yourself.'

This 'enlightenment', the 'returning to the source' and the recovery of our authenticity, are referred to less mystically in our own culture, which has the advantage of making it seem less elusive, more attainable. Abraham Maslow called it 'self-actualization', and listed the characteristics of self-actualizers. These included:

spontaneity, simplicity, naturalness
acceptance of oneself, others and nature
deeper and more profound interpersonal relations
self-actualizing creativeness
detachment and need for privacy
autonomy, independence of culture and environment
continued freshness of appreciation
philosophical, unhostile sense of humour.

Jung talked of 'the individuation process' and suggested that unless we go on developing, and start living at a less superficial level in the second half of life, we are in for trouble. He came to the conclusion that his middle-aged patients had become neurotic because their rigid and conditioned conscious attitudes cut them off effectively from dialogue with their unconscious, and especially its 'religious function', which meant exploring unlived potential, repressed energies, finding meaning in life and coming to terms with death. Many of Jung's patients were outwardly wealthy and successful, yet inside felt arid. Working on the individuation process, exploring their unconscious world of dreams, archetypes and disowned subpersonalities gradually freed their blocked psychic energies, like a river that had been dammed and then began to flow again. This too is the experience of many meditators: that the 'way out' of feeling stale, in a rut, at a dead end, is in fact the 'way in' – searching inside our self for new directions and where our true creativity (vocation?) lies. And the miracle is that when we start to ask the right questions the unconscious always, sooner or later, comes up with the right answers.

WHO AM I?
This is the basic question, for virtually everything we think, feel, say or do arises from who we think we are. Our conditioning, as we have said, is like a straitjacket, confining us only to well-defined, limited ways of moving and being in the world. Whole areas of experiencing, relating, creativity and self-expression are effectively barred to us by our identification with class, nationality, political bias, gender. Gurdjieff used to tell the story of the tiger who thought he was a goat. Brought up by goats, he behaved like a goat – until another tiger one day picked him up by the scruff of the neck and forced him to look at his own reflection in a river. Whereupon

the ex-goat realized his true identity and let out a mighty roar. To realize who we truly are is a relief and a joy – and *empowering*. Especially, as in the case of the Ugly Duckling, when we don't fit in. Experiencing yourself as a square peg in a round hole, having trouble conforming to the expectations of those around you, can be painful and lonely. But it is also a powerful spur to emancipation since it forces you to look within.

Meditation is liberating. It makes us see the relativity of worldly values and find our own authentic style instead of slavishly following current trends and fashions. We become more independent-thinking, open-minded, more tolerant of the pictures that minds other than our own are projecting, simply because we are prepared to allow them the freedom we claim for ourselves. We become our own men and women, self-directing, 'in the world but not of it'. And when you know who you are, you cannot easily be manipulated.

The question 'Who am I?' is the ultimate meditation technique. For Ramana Maharshi, indeed, it was the only one necessary. Before you launch yourself into this inquiry that will take you deeper and deeper into who you really are it could be useful to 'clear the decks' with the following exercise used in Psychosynthesis.

DISIDENTIFICATION EXERCISE

Repeat to yourself the following disidentification, giving yourself time to allow them to sink in.

I am not my body. I am aware of my body. Therefore I cannot be my body.

I am not my feelings. I am aware of my feelings. Therefore I cannot be my feelings.

I am not my thoughts. I am aware of my thoughts. Therefore I cannot be my thoughts.

MEDITATION 20: WHO AM I?

TECHNIQUE

Ask yourself the question 'Who am I'? over and over again. Address the question to your subconscious rather than to your conscious mind. The latter will want to come up with pat answers like your name, what you do for a living – the sort of 'social' answers we would give to a similar query at a party, for example. Reject these answers from the mind ('*neti, neti*' – 'not this, not this') and go on repeating the question. Allow yourself to feel a response, rather than to come up with an intellectual formula.

Eventually the question will begin to feel like a mantra, or a hammer with which you are trying to break down some dimly-felt barrier between you and the answer. And indeed this is exactly what you will be doing: hammering away at your conditioning to find the real you buried underneath.

'Who am I?' in fact is like the koans used by zen masters with their pupils – a device to cut through the 'thinking about' of the mind and reach the level of fresh, spontaneous and direct experience. Coming up with an answer that can be verbalized is not as important as the heightened sense of self that you experience as you discard all the masks behind which you have been taught to hide. Gestalt therapy is one of the modern approaches to personal growth that is very meditative, not least in its insistence on present-centred awareness. Its founder, Fritz Perls, charted the various layers of personality and conditioning that we have to cut through before we can experience being 'real' and authentic again. These layers are roughly what happens when we wrestle with the question 'Who am I?'

Layer 1: the 'cliché' layer, or the layer of token existence. This is the level we operate on when we exchange polite social pleasantries like 'Nice weather we're having' and formal greetings.

Layer 2: The 'role' or 'game-playing' layer. This is the layer in which we pretend to be always a certain type of person, to live up to our own self-image and others' expectations, e.g. 'good', 'kind', 'successful', 'competent', etc.

Layer 3: The 'impasse' layer. When our games and manipulations for whatever reason do not work (as, for example, in therapy) we feel frustrated, 'stuck' with nothingness, for we have lost the props we rely on to get us through life.

Layer 4: The 'implosive' layer. If we can stay with emptiness and uncertainty and resist the temptation to fall back on role-playing, we feel very bleak and almost as if we are dying. It is, in fact, our conditioning, not us that is slipping away.

Layer 5: The 'explosive' layer. If we manage to stay with the 'implosive layer' long enough, eventually we will break through to a level of authentic self-expression. This may manifest initially in areas of 'unfinished business' where we have been blocking the free flow of our energies. Thus we may experience previously unexpressed grief, or the unblocking of sexual energy, or the capacity to feel and express anger, or simply an explosion of joy.

There is a marked correlation between Perls's analysis of what happens when the client's attempts to manipulate the therapist are continually frustrated and reflected back, and the experience of zen meditators wrestling with koans similar to 'Who am I?' (which would probably be set by a zen master in the form of 'Show me your original face before your parents were born'). Before you embark on this quest for yourself you should perhaps read Philip Kapleau's classic *The Three Pillars of Zen* (Boston: Beacon Press, 1965) and decide whether you are ready for this one, for it is the most rigorous of all meditation techniques. By contrast, the next meditation is one of the easiest.

MEDITATION 21: 'THIRD EYE' MEDITATION

TECHNIQUE

Focus on the space between the eyebrows.

Put on a tape of suitable 'meditation music' and turn down the lights. Since this meditation is always done with the eyes open, it is a help to have something pleasing and calming to rest your eyes on. (Raja yoga uses a mandala.) Make sure you are sitting in a comfortable position that you can maintain for half an hour.

Focus attention on your 'third eye' as if you were looking out through it. Do not meditate on anything in particular. Staying centred in this chakra is all you have to do.

This meditation used in modern Raja yoga is one of the simplest and most effective techniques for 'getting you there' – i.e. beyond the turmoil of the physical world and centred in your self. For Raja yogins, this true self is the soul. We don't have a soul, we *are* souls. The location of the soul is between the eyebrows, and if we focus our attention on this spot we can experience soul-consciousness straightaway. The soul is the part of us that is eternal. It has always existed and always will. According to Raja yoga, in the intervals between incarnations it rests in the peace of the soul world, which in life it has a memory of and longs for – and can take us there in a flash, for thought transcends time and space. All our misery is due to forgetting who we really are, and identifying instead with 'body consciousness' which can never really satisfy us, and merely stores up karma that has to be paid off sooner or later. Recovering soul-consciousness, remembering who we really are, we experience the peace, bliss and silence that is our true nature.

Once you have started on a path to self-realization, life meets you halfway. 'Ask, and you shall receive. Knock, and it shall be opened to you.' Or, as they say in the East, 'When the disciple is ready, the guru appears.' You will start meeting other people who are also 'working on themselves' and perhaps can take you a bit further along your path by sharing with you what they have learned. If you are stuck along the path in some way, or perhaps have been puzzling over some existential question and are browsing in a bookshop, it often happens (at least to me) that you pick up at random the right book to read next. It is almost as if you home in on it unconsciously, as if it wants to be read. Jung called this phenomenon 'synchronicity', when the universe seems to be supporting your desire to become more conscious, validating your insights and to be saying: 'Yes, you're on the right track.' For, ultimately perhaps, that is what we are all here to do.

The Jesuit scientist and mystic Teilhard de Chardin envisaged the earth as being surrounded by a layer of consciousness that he called the 'nousphere'. The more conscious beings there are on the planet, the deeper this layer becomes. This suggests that when each of us meditates (or otherwise works on ourselves to become more conscious) we are, in our own small way, helping to make this world of ours more conscious, more peaceful, loving and joyful. Our thoughts and vibrations, whether positive or negative, add to the sum total of the thought forms currently circulating for better or for worse. They will be picked up by others, for nothing travels faster than thoughts and 'No man is an Island, entire of itself; every man is piece of the Continent, a part of the main.'

There is a general consensus that we are living in a time when 'getting our act together' on a global level is becoming a matter of survival. We can no longer afford to go on living unconscious lives, for time is running out. Whether we think in terms of the Aquarian Age of brotherhood and personal responsibility, or the Diamond Age (in which the earth is purifying itself), or are concerned for human and animal rights, individual freedom, ecology, or simply fear nuclear war, the call to us all is to raise our level of consciousness by becoming more aware. And since the royal road to deepening awareness has always been meditation, it follows that the more meditators we have on this planet, the better will be the quality of our lives.

IT'S NOT THAT SERIOUS!

Enlightenment is about 'lightening up'. As you begin to drop the excess baggage of conditioning, as you begin to gain control of your mind by continually witnessing it, you will allow yourself to be brought down less and less by the 'heavy' thoughts that pop into it from time to time and affect your moods. Used now to watching how thoughts come – and go if you don't cling on to them – you know that, however bleak things may be looking right now, 'This Too Shall Pass'. Centred in your awareness rather than hypno-tized, rabbit-like, by the serpent of thought, you will have the distance necessary to be able to counteract negative thinking (which only makes problems worse) by positive affirmations such as 'It always works out, so it must be working out now'. As you see yourself bouncing back again and again from the knocks life deals you, you learn from those experiences to become more aware of your own con-tribution to creating them. You stop complaining, blaming or otherwise playing victim, because you now know that you are, and always have been, the boss where your own life is concerned. And that you can change things and create what you want, simply by remembering who you really are and taking back your power.

In the East, life is seen as a play, a *leela*. The Supreme Identity of God is perhaps the Joker, and the name of the game 'hide-and-seek'. What He (She? It?) hid was the truth about who we really are, for the fun of finding out again. Unfortunately, we became confused as to what we were supposed to be looking for: was it wealth? success? power? And even more confused when we found these and they weren't it. Unawareness of the game means taking everything very seriously, whereas the whole point of playing a game at all is to *enjoy* it, and ourselves. Of course, the more you put into it the more fun you get out of it. But, underneath all the ups and downs, the yells of triumph and the squeals of anguish, there is the awareness that it's only a game. Forgetting this, taking it too seriously, makes us tense, no fun to play with and bad losers.

As long as our mind computers control us we will always take things, and ourselves, far too seriously. Whether or not, as Rajneesh said, 'Seriousness is a Disease', we have seen that the anxiety, tension and stress that it engenders can in fact help to *cause* disease in our bodies. And the reverse, happily, is also true, that enjoying yourself is the best therapy. As far back as the second century A.D., Galen had observed that it was depressed women who got breast cancer, not cheerful ones. That 'laughter is the best medicine' is at last beginning to be taken seriously by the medical profession (at least in the French-speaking world) was shown by a symposium held in Toronto in 1986 for doctors, nurses and therapists. The subject was 'The Healing Power of Laughter'. French researchers have found that laughers are less prone to ulcers and other digestive disorders. According to Dr Pierre Dacher, laughter improves circulation, speeds tissue healing and stabilizes many bodily functions.

Laughing is *good* for you, as Norman Cousins tells us in his best-seller *Anatomy of an Illness*. Crippled with an 'incurable' and very painful disease of the body's connective tissues called ankylosing spondylitis, he had been given a one in 500 chance of survival. Eventually he decided that the twenty-six aspirins and twelve phenylbutazone a day were not doing him much good. Instead, he started taking massive doses of vitamin C and sent out for 'Candid Camera' videos and old Marx Brothers films. Henceforth he spent his day just 'hanging out' and chortling over the films – and healed himself.

Beware of taking anything – including meditation – too

seriously. You can be sincere, and regular in your practice, without being serious. Enjoy your meditation sessions, relax into them. And if you find yourself straining to 'do it right', getting depressed with and repeatedly thrown by the bucking bronco that is your mind, and wanting to give up, you could give yourself a break with the following meditation that was a favourite with Alan Watts.

MEDITATION 22: LAUGHING MEDITATION

TECHNIQUE

Just laugh. At first laughter may not want to come — especially if you are feeling dreadful. But 'just do it' and, by and by, your laughter will become real. (It may help to look at your own doleful expression in a mirror, and to pull some funny faces.) Laugh till the tears roll down your cheeks, until you are giving yourself a bellyache. Then not only will you be doing something only we humans can do, but you will be like Hotei, the Laughing Buddha.

SOME TAPES SUITABLE FOR MEDITATION

Anything by Deuter or Kitaro.
Frank Lorentzen: *Hands*
Kim Menzer/Lars Trier: *Skywalks*
Flemming Petersen: *Moonwater, Airdance, Between Heartbeats*
Mike Rowlands: *Fairy Ring, Silver Wings*
Shardad: *Dream Images* (Search for Serenity Series)
David Sun: *Tranquillity*

These are only a few the author has used and enjoyed. As New Age music becomes more popular, more and more tapes appear which are suitable for use in meditation. The best thing is to ask to hear some before you buy. You can do this, for example, at Mysteries, 9 Monmouth Street, Covent Garden, London WC2.

Flemming Petersen's tapes are available from Fonix Musik, Sonder Alle, 800 Arhus C, Denmark. The Search for Serenity Series is distributed by Inner Harmonies, 3 Crail View, Northleach, Gloucestershire GL54 3QH.

As well as these New Age tapes, tapes of environmental sounds (especially of the sea or running water) can be very soothing, e.g. 'Slow Ocean' and 'Temple in the Forest' (obtainable at Mysteries).

INDEX

FOR THE BEST IN PAPERBACKS, LOOK FOR THE 🐧

In every corner of the world, on every subject under the sun, Penguin represents quality and variety – the very best in publishing today.

For complete information about books available from Penguin – including Puffins, Penguin Classics and Arkana – and how to order them, write to us at the appropriate address below. Please note that for copyright reasons the selection of books varies from country to country.

In the United Kingdom: Please write to *Dept E.P., Penguin Books Ltd, Harmondsworth, Middlesex, UB7 0DA.*

If you have any difficulty in obtaining a title, please send your order with the correct money, plus ten per cent for postage and packaging, to *PO Box No 11, West Drayton, Middlesex*

In the United States: Please write to *Dept BA, Penguin, 299 Murray Hill Parkway, East Rutherford, New Jersey 07073*

In Canada: Please write to *Penguin Books Canada Ltd, 2801 John Street, Markham, Ontario L3R 1B4*

In Australia: Please write to the *Marketing Department, Penguin Books Australia Ltd, P.O. Box 257, Ringwood, Victoria 3134*

In New Zealand: Please write to the *Marketing Department, Penguin Books (NZ) Ltd, Private Bag, Takapuna, Auckland 9*

In India: Please write to *Penguin Overseas Ltd, 706 Eros Apartments, 56 Nehru Place, New Delhi, 110019*

In the Netherlands: Please write to *Penguin Books Netherlands B.V., Postbus 195, NL–1380AD Weesp*

In West Germany: Please write to *Penguin Books Ltd, Friedrichstrasse 10–12, D–6000 Frankfurt/Main 1*

In Spain: Please write to *Longman Penguin España, Calle San Nicolas 15, E–28013 Madrid*

In Italy: Please write to *Penguin Italia s.r.l., Via Como 4, I-20096 Pioltello (Milano)*

In France: Please write to *Penguin Books Ltd, 39 Rue de Montmorency, F-75003 Paris*

In Japan: Please write to *Longman Penguin Japan Co Ltd, Yamaguchi Building, 2–12–9 Kanda Jimbocho, Chiyoda-Ku, Tokyo 101*

PENGUIN HEALTH

Healing Nutrients   Patrick Quillin

A guide to using the vitamins and minerals contained in everyday foods to fight off disease and promote well-being: to prevent common ailments, cure some of the more destructive diseases, reduce the intensity of others, augment conventional treatment and speed up healing.

Total Relaxation in Five Steps   Louis Proto

With Louis Proto's Alpha Plan you can counteract stress, completely relaxing both mind and body, in just 30 minutes a day. By reaching the Alpha state – letting the feelings, senses and imagination predominate – even the most harassed can feel totally rejuvenated.

Aromatherapy for Everyone   Robert Tisserand

The use of aromatic oils in massage can relieve many ailments and alleviate stress and related symptoms.

Spiritual and Lay Healing   Philippa Pullar

An invaluable new survey of the history of healing that sets out to separate the myths from the realities.

Hypnotherapy for Everyone   Dr Ruth Lever

This book demonstrates that hypnotherapy is a real alternative to conventional healing methods in many ailments.

FOR THE BEST IN PAPERBACKS, LOOK FOR THE 🐧

PENGUIN HEALTH

Positive Smear Susan Quilliam

A 'positive' cervical smear result is not only a medical event but an emotional event too: one which means facing up to issues surrounding your sexuality, fertility and mortality. Based on personal experiences, Susan Quilliam's practical guide will help every woman meet that challenge.

Medicine The Self-Help Guide
Professor Michael Orme and Dr Susanna Grahame-Jones

A new kind of home doctor – with an entirely new approach. With a unique emphasis on self-management, *Medicine* takes an *active* approach to drugs, showing how to maximize their benefits, speed up recovery and minimize dosages through self-help and non-drug alternatives.

Defeating Depression Tony Lake

Counselling, medication and the support of friends can all provide invaluable help in relieving depression. But if we are to combat it once and for all we must face up to perhaps painful truths about our past and take the first steps forward that can eventually transform our lives. This lucid and sensitive book shows us how.

Freedom and Choice in Childbirth Sheila Kitzinger

Undogmatic, honest and compassionate, Sheila Kitzinger's book raises searching questions about the kind of care offered to the pregnant woman – and will help her make decisions and communicate effectively about the kind of birth experience she desires.

Care of the Dying Richard Lamerton

It is never true that 'nothing more can be done' for the dying. This book shows us how to face death without pain, with humanity, with dignity and in peace.

PENGUIN HEALTH

Living with Asthma and Hay Fever   John Donaldson

For the first time, there are now medicines that can prevent asthma attacks from taking place. Based on up-to-date research, this book shows how the majority of sufferers can beat asthma and hay fever and lead full and active lives.

Anorexia Nervosa   R. L. Palmer

Lucid and sympathetic guidance for those who suffer from this disturbing illness, and for their families and professional helpers, given with a clarity and compassion that will make anorexia more understandable and consequently less frightening for everyone involved.

Medicines: A Guide for Everybody   Peter Parish

This sixth edition of a comprehensive survey of all the medicines available over the counter or on prescription offers clear guidance for the ordinary reader as well as invaluable information for those involved in health care.

Pregnancy and Childbirth   Sheila Kitzinger

A complete and up-to-date guide to physical and emotional preparation for pregnancy – a must for all prospective parents.

The Penguin Encyclopaedia of Nutrition   John Yudkin

This book cuts through all the myths about food and diets to present the real facts clearly and simply. 'Everyone should buy one' – *Nutrition News and Notes*

The Parents' A to Z   Penelope Leach

For anyone with children of 6 months, 6 years or 16 years, this guide to all the little problems involved in their health, growth and happiness will prove reassuring and helpful.

End galley

PENGUIN HEALTH

Audrey Eyton's F-Plus Audrey Eyton

'Your short cut to the most sensational diet of the century' – *Daily Express*

Baby and Child Penelope Leach

A beautifully illustrated and comprehensive handbook on the first five years of life. 'It stands head and shoulders above anything else available at the moment' – Mary Kenny in the *Spectator*

Woman's Experience of Sex Sheila Kitzinger

Fully illustrated with photographs and line drawings, this book explores the riches of women's sexuality at every stage of life. 'A book which any mother could confidently pass on to her daughter – and her partner too' – *Sunday Times*

Food Additives Erik Millstone

Eat, drink and be worried? Erik Millstone's hard-hitting book contains powerful evidence about the massive risks being taken with the health of the consumer. It takes the lid off food and the food industry.

Living with Allergies Dr John McKenzie

At least 20% of the population suffer from an allergic disorder at some point in their lives and this invaluable book provides accurate and up-to-date information about the condition, where to go for help, diagnosis and cure – and what we can do to help ourselves.

Living with Stress Cary L. Cooper, Rachel D. Cooper and Lynn H. Eaker

Stress leads to more stress, and the authors of this helpful book show why low levels of stress are desirable and how best we can achieve them in today's world. Looking at those most vulnerable, they demonstrate ways of breaking the vicious circle that can ruin lives.